FROM PSYCHING UP TO DEALING WITH SLIP UPS, THIS IS THE ONLY BOOK THAT GIVES YOU A COMPLETE PROGRAM FOR SOLVING YOUR MOST DIFFICULT EATING PROBLEM

⋘ ⋙

Registered nutritionist and dietary consultant Kathy Stone draws on the latest research and her own twenty-year eating battle to offer this unique interactive work for solving the most difficult dilemma for any dieter: getting over those late-night, out-of-control munchies. *Snack Attack* shows how to:

- Cut the fat intake from your snacking to 6 grams or less per day
- Choose the right snacks to satisfy your cravings
- Use visualization exercises to overcome your most difficult eating challenges
- Learn to take failure in stride—so one slip-up will not ruin your diet
- Use a support person or "sponsor" to help you stay in control of your eating habits.

Featuring a remarkable thirty-day schedule, interactive checklists, and coaching and advice designed to help you maintain good eating habits, *Snack Attack* is for every fitness-conscious person who has ever had a problem with the midnight munchies—and who is looking for better health and a truly vibrant sense of self.

S0-DVD-411

SNACK ATTACK

30 DAYS TO CONQUER CRAVINGS

KATHY STONE

WARNER BOOKS

A Time Warner Company

WARNER BOOKS EDITION

Cover photo by Arron Rezny
Cover design by Anne Twomey
Book design by H. Roberts

Warner Books, Inc.
666 Fifth Avenue
New York, N.Y. 10103

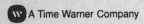 A Time Warner Company

Printed in the United States of America

First Printing: August, 1991

10 9 8 7 6 5 4 3 2 1

Contents

Contents

Introduction

What is a snack attack? Chances are you already know, even if you can't define it in words. I believe it is that irrepressible urge to nibble on everything and anything in the house at nonmeal times. To millions of dieters, it means failure. After counseling people in weight loss for more than ten years and a lifetime of battling my own weight problem, I have identified uncontrolled nibbling as the single most difficult eating pattern to overcome.

Clients who had been successful in eating balanced meals during the day had found that the uncontrollable urge to snack at night was sabotaging their efforts. As a result, they soon felt hopeless and depressed, further damaging their already troubled self-image. These negative feelings made it impossible for them to achieve permanent success. After one night's failure—one candy binge or ice-cream indulgence—they found it difficult to regroup and bring their diets back under control. Furthermore, one deviation from the diet led to more detours from the meal plan, in order to "get all the cravings out of the system," forgetting that all calories must be paid for in some way. A person who is suffering from leftover guilt can't possibly maintain control of his eating habits.

Snack attacks, therefore, often become a cyclical problem; one downfall is followed by another, until the individual gives up entirely. This cycle is particularly devastating to the person who likes to feel in control of his or her life, for failure to maintain a previous day's success begins to erode one's self-confidence, and it creates anger. Because such constant and virtually inevitable failure is so alien to these individuals, they eventually abandon all efforts to stabilize their eating habits.

There is good news, though. You can actually make your snacking habits work for you rather than against you. Coupled with new research in dieting and weight loss, this book will teach you a technique that will make it possible for you to look at dieting in a whole new light, one that ensures success. You'll learn how to do this by following the examples and recommendations in this book, which offer advice on how to permanently change eating habits.

This new pattern of eating, tested successfully with hundreds of clients, modifies snacking rather than tries to eliminate it. In the past, most programs have tried to address weight problems with the same approach as addictions to cigarettes or alcohol are treated. In other words, the "cold turkey" method has been prescribed. That, however, does not work with eating—at least not over the long haul. Of course, there are the short-term successes of the liquid protein diets, even with diets restricted to hot dogs and ice cream. But to attain permanent success and achieve control over eating habits, real lifestyle changes must be implemented, and they must be changes you can live with. Using vinegar mixed with sugar substitute on a salad in place of blue cheese dressing just for the sake of the diet won't do it. The minute the diet ends—in two weeks, on the average—the blue cheese will be back on the salad and the pounds will be back on the dieter.

To control weight and change eating habits, the behavior that drives the eating must be altered permanently. In most cases the bad eating habits have existed for most of the person's life. Such people have never learned to distinguish between true hunger and the desire to eat. Physical hunger is due to a lack of food and is the only legitimate reason to eat. Uncontrolled snacking, however, tends to be based on emotional issues and therefore is a much harder habit to kick.

This book will help you to distinguish between the two kinds of hunger and to react appropriately to each. And, because we live in a fast-paced, results-oriented society, it will teach you to accomplish this in thirty days, with no unhealthy, dangerous gimmicks. You won't be asked to make drastic or impossible changes, just healthy decisions that you can make at a comfortable pace, one step at a time.

By following the daily assignments and helpful hints,

you will master the skills necessary for long-term weight loss and maintenance. Day by day, you will experience a change in your eating habits. Most important, you will know the satisfaction of being in control of your eating again. The outcome will last a lifetime and you will feel terrific.

SNACK ATTACK

What This Book Won't Tell You

What assumptions did you make when you saw the title of this book? Did you think it was going to tell you that the way to control eating was to eat three meals a day and refrain from snacking completely? That's old news!

Recent research has taught us many new and exciting facts that enable us to deal with eating habits more effectively. This is great news, because it means that while you may think you've tried everything, there's new hope.

You may be wondering why it isn't easier just to limit yourself to eating three meals a day. Certainly snacking got you into this situation in the first place. You probably consider nibbling your primary problem, maybe your *only* problem. Your meals likely consist of small, balanced, controlled portions. Snacking, on the other hand, feels wildly uncontrolled—and that can make you feel bad about yourself.

This book will not tell you to eat three meals a day. In fact, it will tell you to eat at least five times per day. It will even go so far as to say that the more often you eat, the better you will look and feel.

When it comes to snacking, research shows us that small, frequent meals are actually better metabolized by the body than are fewer larger meals. You are probably familiar with studies analyzing two groups of people in which one group eats one meal a day that contains 500 calories. The other group eats three meals a day totaling 1,000 calories. Using the accepted theory that when you have eliminated 3,500 calories from your diet, you will lose 1 pound, you would expect that the group consuming half the calories (the 500-calorie group) would lose twice as much weight, twice as fast, than the 1,000-calorie group. In reality, the two groups lose the same amount of weight at the same rate.

This proves that the more frequently meals are eaten, the better they are metabolized. It can be likened to stoking a fire: small amounts of food eaten often burn better. It is also theorized that the body can handle only so many calories at one time; the excess calories are dumped in the fat-storage system. Research does not tell us what this optimal calorie amount is, nor is it likely to be the same amount for each person. However, it does suggest that skipping breakfast and lunch and having one good meal is not the most efficient way to lose weight. Nor will it help you to change your eating habits permanently. In fact, the body may be so resistant to the low-calorie diet that it will lower the metabolism in a compensation mechanism, preventing any significant weight loss. So even though you may cut your daily caloric intake, you may still not lose weight.

The group study also shows that calories are not always equal. We have always thought that if someone cut down to a certain calorie level, he would lose weight. Now we know that he may actually be able to lose weight by eating more calories than first thought, by adjusting *when* the calories are consumed. For example, if you have ever tried dieting by consuming one meal a day of 500 calories, you probably remember that it was not easy. Chances are you felt a great deal of hunger. On the other hand, eating 1,000 calories a day, divided into three or four meals, provides adequate nourishment and is not overly problematic on a long-term basis, if done correctly. The old adage of eating breakfast like a king, lunch like a prince, and dinner like a pauper is more than just an old wives' tale. There is some truth behind the saying. Just ask yourself how active you are during the day as opposed to at night. Most people are at least somewhat active during the day and considerably more sedentary at night. That means the body's metabolism slows down at night and therefore fewer calories are burned.

Now you know why this book will not tell you to eat three meals a day. Nor will it provide you with a long list of forbidden foods.

There aren't any no-no's here. Traditional diet books contain lists of foods that you are not supposed eat. This is because they are *diet* books. This, however, is not a diet book! It will teach you how to modify your behavior and thereby permanently change your eating habits for life. You will learn to control everything you eat.

Not listing foods to avoid will seem foreign to the typical dieter because that person is used to being told what and when to eat and likes it that way. The dieter doesn't want to make decisions, because that implies a certain degree of self-control, which, for the most part, he thinks he doesn't have. In fact, the dieter often doesn't *want* to have self-control, because if he fails on a typical diet, he can blame the diet. On the other hand, if he fails to exhibit self-control, it is he who has failed. It is always harder to blame oneself than to blame other people or circumstances.

As you can see, there is a great deal that this book won't tell you. Furthermore, while this book expects a great deal of you, it asks nothing that you can't do. Assuming that there is still an ounce of control in you and that you are not hopeless (although sometimes you may think you are), you will now learn to analyze and deal with your eating habits in an entirely new way.

Remember that while dieting may help you lose weight, keeping it off is the secret to maintaining a healthy body. Ending uncontrolled snacking will help you accomplish your goals and give you the satisfaction of knowing that *you* did it, not some diet.

Take every chapter literally. Try all the suggestions. You'll want to carry the book with you in order to complete the assignments. This will be helpful because it will enable you to write down your thoughts and feelings while they are fresh in your mind.

At the end of thirty days, you'll find that your control

over food has improved significantly. Then, not only will you look terrific, you'll feel terrific.

Day I Assignment: Write down the assumptions you made when you bought this book. Start carrying it with you wherever you go. It will serve as a workbook for you to learn to change your eating patterns.

WORKSHEET

Initial Assumptions

1. _____
2. _____
3. _____
4. _____
5. _____

Examples:

1. I thought the book would tell me snacking was bad.
2. I thought the book would have a diet plan with lots of recipes.

2

Motivation: It's Time To Psyche Up

Why do you want to gain control of your eating habits and ultimately lose weight? If that seems like a silly question, consider the following silly scenarios.

Will losing weight make you rich? Possibly, but it's doubtful. Will losing weight make your job more satisfying? That depends on what you do or whether losing weight would enable you to change careers, but for most of us, losing weight is fairly independent of job satisfaction. Will gaining control of your eating habits make you feel more in control of all other aspects of your life? Well, many aspects, maybe, but *all* of them . . . ?

As you can see, it is difficult to predict the effects that losing weight will have on your life. But it is vitally important to recognize which reasons for wanting to lose weight are valid and which ones are not. Once you have determined this, you will be able to achieve the necessary motivation to change your eating habits.

Do you have a cholesterol problem? Does your weight problem cause you to breathe too heavily when you walk up a flight of stairs? Do you want to look better in your clothes? If the answer to any, or all, of the above is yes, then you have some legitimate reasons for wanting to lose weight. These reasons all concern areas of good health, well-being, and even vanity.

On the other hand, losing weight will not solve your relationship problems with other people. This common assumption among dieters not only is exaggerated but virtually ensures failure. Consider this: You lose weight with the idea that being thinner will solve difficult problems with a friend, spouse, or lover. But once you've achieved your ideal weight, you find that the same problems still exist. Thus, you learn that your main reason for wanting to be thin wasn't valid. You will then find it virtually impossible to keep that weight off. In addition, you will experience depression. Therefore, there is only one person worth changing your behavior for: *you*! Focus on the positive reasons for losing weight and you will experience greater success satisfaction in the end.

The right motivation is an essential part of gaining control of one's eating habits. Right motivation is composed of certain mental images that need to be deeply embedded in the mind when the temptation times roll around. Intentions are terrific, but of themselves they do not produce success; if they did, we would all have the control we wanted in all aspects of our lives.

When beginning to build up the right motivation, ask yourself why this is the right time to gain control of your eating. Your answer may be, *It's not the right time*. In fact, usually it is not the right time. There's always some special event, or company, or social function coming up, at which you anticipate eating in an uncontrolled manner; therefore, you think maybe it would be best to wait. *Wrong!*

First of all, there is no better time than now to get on with the rest of your life in a more positive mode. Second, there is always an excuse for deciding that this is not a good time. And reasoning that this is not a good time is based on black-and-white thinking.

The theory most widely believed by dieters is that if they do not perfectly follow their diets, they are total failures. Many negative behaviors are associated with such thinking. For example, how many times have you "blown it" on a diet by eating a larger than permitted portion and then felt guilty because you cheated? Instead of resolving to do better, you probably said, "Oh well, I blew it, so I might as well get all my cravings out of my system." You then proceeded to eat everything in sight, all the while vowing to get back on track tomorrow. But how could you? You still harbored the original guilt that started the binge, in addition to your guilt over the binge itself. The result of so much compounded guilt is that it becomes almost impossible to start anew.

Therefore, it is vital not to think in terms of perfection or failure, or to live with a black-and-white mentality. You can do this if you continue to remind yourself that you are not dieting. Rather, you are teaching yourself a new approach to eating. You must learn to live in the gray zone. When you're not happy with the way you just ate, take it in stride, don't beat yourself up for it, and go forward positively.

Pictures can be great motivators for some people. If you have a picture of yourself when you were thinner that you particularly like, carry it with you or tape it to the front of the refrigerator. It will be a constant reminder of what you are trying to achieve and, more important, can achieve. Once you start gaining control and losing weight, carry a picture of yourself at your heaviest. It will reinforce your improved behavior and increased control.

✳ Say positive things to yourself. Make up little sayings or affirmations that will help you through the tough times. One of the most effective is: **Nothing tastes as good as being thin feels.** This statement often puts things into a clearer perspective.

Frequently, people list increased life span as a reason for wanting to lose weight. While this is an excellent incentive, for long-term motivation consider that to most people it is the quality of life that is most important. Nobody wants to live to be eighty years old if his last twenty years were spent wishing he were dead because his body was in such sad shape. Gaining control of your eating patterns will have long-term positive effects both physically and mentally.

Consider all motivators discussed in this chapter and continue to add to your list daily. These personal motivators will provide a strong foundation for achieving your goals. From there it's a piece of cake! Oh, *sorry!*

Day 2 Assignment: Write down ten reasons why it is important for you to gain control of your eating habits and lose weight. Think of controlling your eating habits as the most important aspect. When this is achieved, the weight will melt away permanently.

Make a point of reading these ten reasons each day. Every time you have a desire to eat inappropriately, take out this list and read it! Read it out loud if you can, and read every word. This list shows how you attained your initial "right motivation" and will serve as your mainstay throughout the retraining phase, which lasts thirty days. Maintaining motivation is sometimes difficult, so keep the book with you and read your list. Now, write the list!

WORKSHEET

Ten Reasons I Want to Gain Control of My Eating Habits and Lose Weight

1. _____

2. _____

3. _____

4. _____

5. _____

6. _____

7. _____

8. _____

9. _____

10. _____

Examples:

1. Good: To feel better physically (okay, but not specific
   enough)
   Better: To stop panting when I walk
2. Good: To have my clothes fit better (okay, but you
   know what your real goal is)
   Better: To fit into my old size-12 clothes
3. Good: To work on my cholesterol level
   Better: To reduce my cholesterol to under 200

3

I Eat Because . . .

f you ask people why they eat, most will tell you they eat because they're hungry. When you question them more specifically, they will admit that they eat for a variety of reasons that have little or nothing to do with hunger. For each of the reasons—boredom, anxiety, happiness, sadness—there is a different solution to bring eating habits under control. For example, if boredom is the cause of eating inappropriately, then getting out of the house and involved in nonfood-related activities may be the first step to a solution.

Many people think hunger and appetite are the same thing, but this is not the case. Essentially, appetite is psychological and hunger is physical. It can be extremely difficult to distinguish between them, so let's let's examine each.

Appetite is the brain's response to the senses that are used during eating. When we get up from the dinner table and see a commercial on TV for a decadent piece of chocolate cake and our stomachs start to growl, we wonder how we could possibly be hungry. The answer is, we're not. It's all in our heads. Our eyes see the cake and transmit a signal to our brains that tells us it is time to eat something we adore. The brain then sends a signal to the stomach to produce more gastric acid because it is time to eat, and the extra acid makes the stomach growl. This is a physiological response to a mental image that results in a physical symptom. Such complexities can leave you barely able to distinguish psychological hunger from true hunger without analyzing each situation and how it occurred.

Therefore, it is necessary to look at what triggers the desire to eat over and above your planned meals and snacks in order to determine the difference between hunger and appetite. Certain situations precede our overeating, and at those times we tend to go for high-fat foods. These situations can be called triggers.

Let's look at some of them. For now we will learn to identify them. Later in the book, we will develop strategies to deal with triggers.

BOREDOM. This is probably the biggest cause of snack attacks. It is the old "couch potato" syndrome. Americans spend too much time in front of the television, and that has been linked to overeating due to more influence by advertisements and less exercise due to sitting on the butt! The typical scenario is to watch TV, then get up at commercial time and gaze into the refrigerator until you find something that looks appealing to eat.

ANXIETY/NERVOUSNESS. This trigger can affect

appetite in either direction. Some people will swear that this is the number-one cause of their unplanned snacking. Others will tell you that in periods of extreme anxiety, they are unable to eat. The most important consideration here is that while occasional anxiety may trigger appetite change, some people are chronically nervous or anxious, which may drive their eating behavior continuously.

DEPRESSION. This may be a chronic or occasional situation and may even result from prior inappropriate eating. The use of food to fill the sense of emptiness that accompanies depression is common.

SLEEPLESSNESS/FATIGUE. When you are frequently fatigued, you often do not possess the energy, the mental edge, to fight the battle against overeating. Chapter 4 will discuss the theory that some people are more prone than others to overeating. If this theory is accepted, then it must also be accepted that to control one's overeating will always be a struggle. In such cases, it takes enormous mental and physical energy to fight the battle.

ANGER/FIGHTING. A fight with a loved one or an employer can cause you to raid the kitchen pantry. It is better to be prepared with alternative coping behaviors, because we all know that such behaviors will happen again.

In trying to analyze why we eat, we must realize that there is no easy answer. In many instances, people have asked me why they can't just take a diet pill. The above examples show that psychological/emotional factors have more to do with eating, especially nibbling, than does true physical hunger. Therefore, a pill will not control those signals that the senses send to the brain. Also, pills are not a permanent solution to the problem.

In a final attempt to determine whether you are truly hungry, ask yourself the following:

Has it been more than three hours since I last ate?

Have I missed a meal today?

Can I say that there has not been a visible trigger to my appetite?

Is there some unusual reason why I might be hungry?

If the answer to two or more of these questions is yes, you are probably legitimately hungry. More important, though, is that even if all your answers are no, if you take the time to ask yourself these questions every time you want to eat at an unplanned time, you'll likely talk yourself out of eating at half of those times. And this would be an improvement over your current behavior.

Day 3 Assignment: Using the form below, record when and what you eat today because you think you are really hungry. If you are not sure whether you are truly hungry, mark that too. Maybe a few days from now you'll be able to determine better. This is one area where practice definitely helps.

WORKSHEET

I Think I Was Really Hungry and I Ate:

7:00	3:00
8:00	4:00
9:00	5:00
10:00	6:00
11:00	7:00
12:00	8:00
1:00	9:00
2:00	10:00
	11:00

I Think Something Else Triggered My Appetite and I Ate:

7:00	3:00
8:00	4:00
9:00	5:00
10:00	6:00
11:00	7:00
12:00	8:00
1:00	9:00

2:00   10:00

                              11:00

Examples:

I Think I Was Really Hungry and I Ate:

9:00 *Breakfast:* 2 pieces toast and 8 oz. skim milk—ate because I was hungry, hadn't eaten since 9 P.M. last night.

I Think Something Else Triggered My Appetite and I Ate:

2:30 P.M. Had words with my boss and grabbed a candy bar.

4

Excuses

Now that we've discussed some of the reasons for inappropriate eating and how to tell the difference between hunger and appetite, let's explore the excuses for overeating. Some are legitimate, some are not. The not-legitimate ones vary from social activities that revolve around food to a family that likes to keep junk food in the house. The legitimate reasons for overeating include a family history of obesity and the concept of some people being "born eaters."

My friend Debbie is the perfect example of someone who is not a born eater. Like myself, Debbie was trained as a dietitian, but unlike me, she does not practice in the counseling field—thank goodness! Debbie is 5 feet 9 inches tall and weighs 130 pounds (in other words, she is very, very thin). Debbie will tell you that she watches her weight, but the truth is, she really doesn't care as much for eating as do people who have weight problems.

For example, we went to the beach one Saturday and Debbie brought a can of potato chips. Now, potato chips are not among my usual binge foods, but I could get into trouble with them out of boredom. I will always have to watch what I eat. Abstaining from unscrupulous snacking will never come naturally and I accept that. On this particular day, Debbie opened the potato chips, took out a few, and then placed them as close to my chair as she could without saying a word. I was acutely aware of her actions but said nothing. I waited for about ten minutes, then took out a few chips and, without saying a word, placed the can back next to her chair. At that point Debbie said, "I was offering them to you," to which I replied, "Thank you, I had a few and now I'm returning them to you."

Debbie then reminded me that we were going skiing together in three weeks and said, "I hope you're not on one of your silly diets when we're on vacation because I eat Cadbury bars and M&Ms when I'm on vacation." I replied, "Listen, your idea of eating M&Ms is that you buy a pound and it lasts you a week. My idea of eating M&Ms is I buy a pound and it lasts me maybe an hour!"

And that's the way it is. There isn't *always* an underlying reason for overeating. I believe some of us were born that way.

Others truly do have underlying psychological reasons, and some of these will be briefly discussed here. If you find yourself in the following scenarios, this book, because of its emphasis on behavior analysis, will still be a great help to you. Keep in mind, however, that some problems do require professional psychological intervention.

In the previous chapters we discussed the fallacy that being thin will solve relationship problems. But often the opposite can be true: a person has very low self-esteem and overeats in order to create a barrier between himself and others. In doing so, he reinforces his poor opinion of himself because he makes himself undesirable to be around.

Other psychological reasons for overeating include a previous lack of emotional support from parents, which leads to a dependence on food for the comfort it provides, and to the use of food as a control issue, in which it becomes the one element over which the person has any control.

Sometimes genetic factors may play a part in a person's being overweight. Several studies have been conducted in which fraternal twins who were adopted at birth were followed for development of obesity in later years. They found that children born to thin parents and placed with overweight adoptive families remained thin. They also showed that children born to overweight parents and placed with thin adoptive parents remained or became overweight. This essentially negates the environmental theory of obesity, which advocates that children become fat because they observe their parents' poor eating habits and because they have increased access to a greater amount of fatty foods.

Unfortunately, if you have genetic tendencies toward

obesity, you're going to have to try even harder to perfect your eating behavior. Fortunately you *can* learn to do this.

There are also social excuses for overeating. In fact, they often explain why we end up eating more calories during the evening meal, when we need the least amount of calories. Dinner is still the most social meal, and many people have a lot of social and professional dinner commitments. The temptation to overeat is great while one's mind is preoccupied with concerns other than the types and amounts of food one is consuming.

There are also the extenuating circumstances of traveling and dining out, and special occasions such as holidays, birthdays, and so on. Social eating makes controlled eating more difficult, for the temptations are greater and the foods are generally prepared with more calories than they would be at home.

As I stated earlier, there seems never to be a "right time" to tackle these excuses. One can always find a reason to put off learning to control his or her eating. The first thing you must do is decide what is important, and if controlling your eating is a priority, then your excuses are mere justifications and their validity diminishes.

Now it is time to examine the excuses you have used in the past and evaluate them on a new level. If you learned bad eating habits from your parents, you will need to learn new, better ones. If you find yourself in many social eating situations, you must learn when to say "when." If you believe you are destined to be fat because of genetics, you need to learn new ways to stimulate your metabolism. In order to learn these things, first you must face them on paper, in black and white, and then you can deal with them in the manner most appropriate for you.

Day 4 Assignment: Refer to the following worksheet. Record what you think triggers your snack attacks (see examples provided), *plus* whether any one particular trigger creates a desire for different foods or if the desire is always for the same foods.

It is important to recognize these triggers so that you can learn to stop justifying your current behavior. Then it is important to memorize words integral to breaking all addictions:

> **God, grant me the serenity**
> **To accept the things I cannot change,**
> **The courage to change the things I can,**
> **And the wisdom to know the difference.**

After writing down what triggers your appetite, recite the above and do so every time you are faced with a difficult eating decision.

WORKSHEET

What Triggers My Appetite:

1. _____
2. _____

3. _____
4. _____

Examples:

1. After dinner: nothing special, I just want to eat **sweets** at night.

2. Food commercials on television: especially for baked foods and pizza; I crave the foods I see.

3. The smell of spicy food or baked goods—I crave the food I think I smell.

5

How to Stop Walking Unconsciousness

An awareness of what and how much you eat on a daily basis may seem like basic knowledge to you. However, chances are strong that you are not aware of much of what you eat. When I was a waitress in college and always trying to diet, I would never have dreamed of eating a plate of french fries. "Too fattening," I would have said. What I seemed never to be aware of was that in the course of a night of waitressing, whenever a french fry dropped from a plate onto my tray, I would eat it! On any given evening, I easily could have eaten two plates of french fries, and then to top it off at the end of the evening, I would say to myself, "Gee, I haven't eaten dinner tonight." In reality I had consumed several hundreds of "unconscious calories." I would then, of course, proceed to eat a meal at eleven o'clock at night.

Another example of our lack of awareness is what I call *walking unconsciousness*. This is the period of time in a dieter's year that usually begins around Thanksgiving and ends around Valentine's Day.

People usually start diets sometime in early or midsummer, perhaps because it is bathing-suit season, or because they want to feel lighter during the hot months. Thanksgiving provides the first big control test to the dieter. Whether he does well at controlling his eating may well set the tone for future success or failure. Because, as we all know, there are many more tests right around the corner. There are the holiday parties of December, the holiday itself, and then of course New Year's, and ultimately Valentine's Day. The whole test time lasts about three months. During it, a few key behavior changes occur.

The most obvious behavior change is that control of eating diminishes. But the supporting behaviors that change are even more important. Such behavior changes are called *The Foundation* and will be discussed in later chapters, but here is one example of such a behavior change. A person should weigh him- or herself once a week. When a diet is going well, the person wants to weigh himself hourly, but the crucial point here is that during this three-month holiday period the individual forgets to check his weight. Thus, the period of walking unconsciousness begins. The individual knows his eating is out of control, but he doesn't want to get on the scale and see the damage. So he waits and says, "I'll do better next week and then I'll weigh myself because then I won't be so depressed by the results." And of course something happens the following week and he doesn't get back on track and therefore keeps postponing the inevitable weigh-in.

The person knows he must be gaining some weight because his clothes fit a bit tighter. But without the black-and-white confirmation of the scale, he can go on believing it isn't that bad. The loose layers of clothes worn in most parts of the country during this time of the year contribute to this denial.

Finally, in late February he meets up with the scale and faces the facts. The results are bad—much worse than he anticipated. Usually crushed with depression, he finds it virtually impossible to regain control.

There are several behavior changes that could have stopped the bleeding before it became a hemorrhage. The most important aspect of this example is that if the individual had been weighing himself on a weekly basis, there would have been a greater chance of getting back in control before he experienced a total downfall. Stopping before you believe it's too late is a key to staying in control.

Most people will tell you they're aware of what they do that is wrong, they just need policing, or to be able to read it in black and white to make it work. The truth is they are only dimly aware of how great their eating problems are, and until they comprehend the severity of the specific problems, they will never be able to solve them. Therefore, awareness must include monitoring various segments of a problem by breaking that problem down and scrutinizing its parts.

For instance, realizing that uncontrolled eating after dinner is one's primary problem is too broad a statement. It might be stated that the problem is partially that the individual goes into the kitchen too often, and once in there opens the refrigerator door and stares until he finds something that suits his mood. Therefore, monitoring the situation by placing a piece of paper just inside the kitchen entrance and placing a slash mark on the paper each time that person enters the kitchen is the first step toward greater awareness. This should be done for a week before the person attempts to change the behavior, although just monitoring such behavior tends automatically to modify it.

Another way to observe your behavior is to let someone else do it for you. This can be difficult because diet-conscious people tend to be defensive about their eating habits, especially around those with whom they are closest. This will be discussed further in chapter 28, "Support mechanisms."

When and where else does your eating go out of control? A food diary will help you monitor your eating habits. As you start to analyze, remember not to tackle too much at once. Awareness takes a great deal of time to develop. But remember that it is the key to gaining control. So, hone those observation skills!

Day 5 Assignment: Begin keeping a daily food diary. Record everything you eat and drink. Record where you were, whom you were with, and the time of the day. See the examples and form below.

<u>WORKSHEET</u>

Food Diary

FOOD	TIME OF DAY	PLACE	WITH WHOM

Examples:

FOOD	TIME OF DAY	PLACE	WITH WHOM
8 ounces skim milk ¾ cup cornflakes banana coffee with 1 teaspoon sugar	8:30 A.M.	kitchen	alone
ham sandwich 1½ oz bag potato chips 12 ounces soda	1:00 P.M.	deli	co-worker
candy bar = 2 oz	4:00	desk	alone
handful of nuts	5:30	kitchen	alone

SNACK ATTACK

Food	Time of Day	Place	With Whom
½ chicken breast			
½ cup mashed potatoes			
small ear of corn	6:30	table	spouse
2 teaspoons margarine			
salad, with 2 tablespoons dressing			
iced tea with 2 teaspoons sugar			
1 cup of ice cream	8:00	TV room	spouse

6

The 10/90 Rule

*I*n this chapter I will discuss many of the habits that turn people into nibblers. Most people who have weight problems claim that they are in control of their eating habits until about 3:00 P.M. These are people who are breakfast or lunch skippers, or both. These people are almost starving themselves until late afternoon, at which time they completely lose control and go on an eating spree that lasts almost eight hours.

THE 10/90 RULE

Most people awaken at around 7:00 A.M. and retire at about 11:00 P.M. For them, the midpoint of the day is 3:00 P.M. Now, since we should have eaten two out of three meals by 3:00 P.M. (breakfast and lunch), we should have consumed 67 percent (⅔) of our caloric intake by 3:00 P.M.

Even if you never eat breakfast, 3:00 P.M. is still the midpoint of the day, and at least 50 percent of the calories for the day should have been consumed. But if we are not in control of our eating habits we consume only 10 percent of our daily caloric intake by 3:00, and the rest—90 percent—by 11:00 P.M. This is the 10/90 rule.

We have already discussed some of the excuses for such eating habits. Dinner is almost always the heaviest meal of the day. It seems the only time when people are able to sit down together as a family—in great contrast to years past when the farm family had a hearty breakfast and lunch to fortify them with the caloric energy necessary to perform heavy physical labor. They realized that there was no need to eat so heavily at night, before going to bed.

Eating few or no calories early in the day creates many difficulties. Scientific research has now shown us that the more an individual cuts his caloric intake during the day, the more his body perceives the threat of starvation. The body therefore slows its metabolism in anticipation of not receiving adequate food during the rest of the day. What this means is that although the person may be eating fewer calories, he is also burning fewer calories, because his body is hoarding whatever food energy it has been given. Consequently, weight loss is nearly impossible.

Also consider this: no matter how much or how little activity a person engages in during the day, he is inevitably more sedentary in the evening. Thus, fewer calories are utilized. The body literally goes to sleep on them.

We are more likely to skip breakfast than any other meal, claiming that as long as we don't eat we don't get hungry, but if we eat breakfast we feel starved an hour and a half later. The problem with this premise is that skipping meals during the day almost always leads to bingeing at night. Skipping breakfast has also been shown to negatively affect metabolism, which is one of the determining factors in losing weight. To avoid feeling hungry after eating breakfast, eat protein (milk, egg, yogurt, et cetera), which is digested slowly. It is then less likely for you to become hungry sooner. You'll also want to have a planned, midmorning snack, as discussed in chapter 13.

Always remember that skipping meals leads to bingeing.

There is also evidence demonstrating that a body can handle only a certain quantity of calories at any particular time. Calories consumed beyond that amount are not well metabolized and are likely to be converted into stored fat. When a person nibbles continually from 5:00 till 10:00 P.M., the body perceives it as one large meal, since little time has elapsed from dinner through the continual snacks.

The answer to this dilemma is that you must eat more calories during the day and fewer at night until you achieve a 50/50 balance with 3:00 to 5:00 P.M. as the midpoint range of your day (adjust slightly up or down to accommodate your daily waking hours). Chapter 12 provides a balanced meal plan to help you lose weight. It calls for two meals and two snacks to be consumed by 3:00 to 5:00 P.M., which you must eat by the prescribed times, even if you are not hungry.

If you are completely unaccustomed to this, start slowly. We wouldn't want to shock your body or make you sick! But, you must begin to try. Your success is greatly based on this fundamental principle. If you currently never eat breakfast, set a goal of having it three times a week to start. Also, have only the portion we recommend for the first two weeks. By the third week, breakfast should begin to be a natural expectation of your body.

Remember, it's not what you eat as much as *when* you eat!

Day 6 Assignment: Post a piece of paper at the entrance to the kitchen and for twenty-four hours mark an X each time you enter the kitchen. Include every time you go in, even if it is to throw away a piece of trash. It is important for you to be acutely aware of how often you enter the room where your food is stored and prepared.

WORKSHEET

7:00	3:00
8:00	4:00
9:00	5:00
10:00	6:00
11:00	7:00
12:00	8:00
1:00	9:00
2:00	10:00
	11:00

Example:

7:00 XXXX	3:00
8:00	4:00
9:00	5:00 XXXXX XXXXX
10:00	6:00 XXXXX
11:00	7:00 XXXXX XXXX
12:00	8:00 XXX
1:00	9:00 XXXXX XXXX
2:00	10:00 XXX
	11:00 XX

7

Spoon-Feed Me,
I Don't Want
to Make Decisions

How many diets have you tried? Do you feel that you failed the diets, or that the diets failed you? One of the biggest mistakes we make when anticipating a change in eating habits is to expect perfection. As stated earlier, anything else feels like bingeing and is viewed as failure. Once we have made a mistake, we think we are horrible and hopeless, and then we eat more, reinforcing this opinion. Only when someone has eaten each food on a diet exactly as it is printed will he tell you that his diet is going well.

To a certain degree this desire for perfection is compulsive. The majority of people with weight problems also experience compulsiveness in other aspects of their personalities. Eventually, it will be important for you to determine and then regulate any other compulsive behavior patterns you may discover. Your need to do this will stem from the fact that once you gain control of your eating habits, you will want to protect yourself from throwing that energy into some other bad habit. For instance, you would not want to give up eating poorly only to start smoking or to increase your smoking if you already do so.

Such behavior will happen only if you rush the process this book recommends. So, remember that behavioral changes take time. Don't expect quick fixes or perfection. Take it *slowly*!

The statement, "I don't want to make decisions," refers to still another dietary approach. This person feels so out-of-control that he wants to be spoon-fed his diet. Sometimes a client will walk into my office and request that I write a specific diet that gives them no options. They want complete menus for every day of the week and a list of foods they are not allowed to eat. These are also the individuals who often consider liquid diets, even if they only have 20 pounds to lose. As you now know, liquid diets are the "cold turkey" approach to losing weight, and this kind of thinking removes temptation only temporarily.

You must learn to make your own food decisions in order to feel you are controlling your weight loss. You will then experience satisfaction and maintain your ideal weight. How to begin making such decisions is not as difficult as you might think.

As I mentioned previously, it is very important to break down behavior into its smallest components when trying to attain solutions. Attempts to change a behavioral pattern that is too complex cannot be successful. The pattern must be simplified and realistic goals developed.

It is also essential to establish a positive base in order to build success. The following provides two examples of how to break down behavioral patterns and begin the decision-making process.

When people come home from work between 4:00 and 6:00 P.M. they frequently have not eaten since lunch at noon or 1:00 P.M. Maybe they even skipped lunch. They then frequently grab all kinds of snacks the minute they walk in the door. They are so hungry that they just can't wait until dinner. Often the calories they consume in nibbling are equivalent to those of a full dinner.

Further complicating matters, this typical nibbling is the beginning of an evening of uncontrolled eating. As cautioned earlier, we need to learn the causes of this behavior. Here are some questions to ask yourself:

Does the snacking happen every night when I get home? If not, what nights does it happen and why?

Does the snacking happen at the same time? Maybe it only happens when I have had a stressful day. Maybe it only happens when I work later than usual.

Does the snacking happen independently of the amount I consumed at lunch? Maybe it only happens when I eat a tossed salad for lunch instead of something more substantial.

These and other questions will give you ideas about how to break down behavior into more specific parts. If you have narrowed the problem down to the fact that your snacking occurs when you arrive at home after a particularly stressful day, then you can start to think of solutions. Here are three suggestions.

1. Drink a diet soda just before going home. This will give you time to relax.

2. Have a snack before leaving the office. This will work only if you can relax there, since the eating is connected not to hunger but to job stress.

3. Go to an aerobics class on the stressful days. Have your gym clothes in the car so you won't need to go straight home. If your family depends on you to be home right after work, try to predict the more stressful days (frequently this *can* be done) and arrange for your family to expect you to be late.

Let's take one more example.

Do you work in an office? Is it one of those offices where goodies are always around? Do doughnuts, crackers, bagels, muffins, cookies, and the monthly birthday celebration keep you snacking uncontrollably? If so, the following will help you determine solutions.

Do you indiscriminately nibble on everything or is it one particular type of food? For instance, is it only sweets that you grab?

Does the snacking take place throughout the day or at a specific time?

Do you snack in front of other people or only when you are alone?

These are key questions that will help you understand what other behavioral patterns are involved with your eating. If you determine that the snacking takes place all through the day and on any food item, not just sweets, try these step-by-step suggestions for solving the problems.

1. Decide to permit yourself to eat the goodies on only two days per week. You will probably think this is still too often, but consider your current situation.

2. Decide to limit the nibbling to only two food items. Pick one that you find the least desirable of the items available and one that you like relatively well, but not your favorite food.

3. Skip all the food items for three weeks except for one small indulgence each day. Make a deal with yourself to bring your own snacks to work for this time period. Then promise yourself a reward at the end of the three weeks if you are 90 percent successful. (Reward systems will be discussed in chapter 22.)

The above examples give a rough idea of how to focus on a problem and then find a solution. In later chapters this process will be further refined and your success in picking the most workable solution will occur more readily.

Day 7 Assignment: Isolate some aspect of your snacking behavior and write three suggestions of how it might begin to be corrected. Take the easiest eating habit even if it seems very unimportant so that you are bound to succeed and feel good about gaining control over this eating habit. As you continue on with this exercise you can choose more difficult scenarios. Think of each solution as being only a temporary answer to the snacking problem, for the solutions will not work all the time. Long-term control of your eating habits requires constant revision whenever necessary.

WORKSHEET

Suggestions to Change One Aspect of Uncontrolled Snacking Behavior:

Problem:

1. _____
2. _____
3. _____

Example:

Suggestions to Change This Aspect

Problem: Snacking on chocolate candy at my desk in the afternoon

1. Take an apple to work to eat instead.
2. Buy a pack of Lifesavers instead of chocolate.

3. Promise yourself a diet chocolate pudding for after-dinner dessert if you don't eat at your desk in the afternoon.

8

Behavioral Change: The Impossible Dream?

Most people have tried to modify their behavior and have failed so many times that they tend to believe it can't be done. The very concept causes fears of failure.

Having been a chronic overeater for most of my life, I know that what behavioral change represents is what repels me most. When I used to think of achieving behavioral change, I thought it meant that I would always be in control of my eating habits and, therefore, able to eat anything I wanted. Ask any chronic overeater if he thinks he will ever be able to eat anything he wants even if he loses all the weight he wants and he will tell you, "No way!" I agree, but only in the short run. Statements about lifetime control are too unrealistic to make and too difficult to attain when an individual is as short-term oriented as most dieters are.

A recent survey stated that despite the fact that most Americans believe that a balanced diet is desirable, they still categorize foods as "good" or "bad." When experts say this is an inappropriate, unbalanced view of foods, they are referring to the person who has no particular tendency to overeat. This book is not targeted at those individuals. As I mentioned earlier, there will always be reasons to fear that normal eating may never be possible because of a long-standing history of abnormal eating. So if behavioral change is in doubt, then what?

Tricks! Learning eating tricks will get a person through the short run. Usually the behavioral change will then kick in by itself later on. I actually *do* believe in and advocate behavioral change, but I know it comes about too slowly for the average dieter. It therefore can't be counted on solely during the initial stages of tackling uncontrolled snacking.

I also will never promote the premise that a person who has always been a chronic nibbler will ever have complete control over his eating habits *with every food*. For example, if chocolate candy is a tremendous weakness for you, then you need to identify that as such and act accordingly. This will take on different meanings for you at different stages of learning to control your eating habits. For instance, when you are first learning to control your craving, chocolate candy is something you should avoid completely. At a more advanced stage, chocolate candy will still be considered a "weakness food" and generally should be avoided. By then you will accept the fact that when you eat chocolate, you likely will still do so in uncontrollable quantities. Hopefully, however, you will have learned to limit the frequency with which you choose to eat candy.

You will always realize that you will probably binge when you eat chocolate, but instead of doing it every week, perhaps you will do it only once a month.

So what are the tricks that will help you through the early stages of changing your eating habits? The following are tricks you should try now!

Remove the majority of the "temptation food" from your house. There was a time in my life when it didn't matter if the food I wanted wasn't in my house at 10:00 P.M. I'd just go out and buy it! But after not having tempting food in the house for a long period of time, I finally got too lazy to go out and buy it. Eventually this will happen to you, but in the meantime . . .

Give your neighbor your car keys. Make a deal with a friend or neighbor to take your keys at the end of the day and not give them back to you until morning. It may sound silly, but it will solve the problem, and you'll gain control in the meantime, so this measure will be necessary only in the short run.

Take a different route. If you drive or walk past a place where you frequently grab a snack that you know is detrimental, go out of your way to avoid that place. Drive three blocks to avoid passing the ice-cream store if necessary. Buy your gas at a place that doesn't have a convenience store attached.

Put all food away in closets, pantries, and so on. Remember my skinny friend Debbie? She has jars of M&Ms and Hershey's Kisses on her kitchen counter. It drives me crazy. I can't do anything about Debbie's counter, but I can keep mine free of distractions. Do you think that won't help—that you'll just remember what's in the closet the next time you have a snack attack? This is a possibility, but I can't tell you how many times that I forgot the temptation foods I had in my closets, even when my cravings were terrible. Of course, if you tend to raid the pantry anyway, you'll have to keep the goodies strictly out of the house.

Eat with a small spoon. Do you use a tablespoon to eat your soup and cereal? Don't! It lets you eat too quickly which is probably one of your problems. The slower you eat, the better you will control your eating. This is just a way of tricking yourself into it.

Make rules. This book contains a number of lifetime rules to live by, but for now let's consider the most difficult to achieve: *to make eating a pure activity*. This means eating without distraction—no television, no reading material, no feeding the kids with one hand or making notes to the baby-sitter with the other. In some respects, this cannot always be accomplished. In our eat-on-the-run society, grabbing food at various times and places is sometimes inevitable. However, it leads to a variety of eating problems and should be avoided. If you are busy at work and have several phone calls to make during lunch, you may decide to eat at your desk while working. You make your phone calls. The next thing you notice is that the second half of your sandwich is gone! It was there a minute ago. You look around, as if wondering who came in and ate your half a sandwich. What happened is that you ate the sandwich without being conscious of doing so. The consequence of this is that you still feel hungry because you did not enjoy eating the lunch that usually fills you up. Therefore, you will probably be tempted to have unplanned snacks later and for the rest of the afternoon.

One more point needs to be made about eating as a pure activity. There is definitely a problem with uncontrolled eating and small-size foods. An example of this is cookies. Without being aware of it, you are likely to eat several cookies at a time because they are small. Since eating is a pure activity, you should consume your meals and snacks at a formal place setting. Relating this to cookies, how much less satisfying do you think cookies are when eaten at the dining-room table rather than in front of the television?

Day 8 Assignment: Choose one of the tricks that you learned in this chapter or make up one of your own. Select a trick that will help you solve an easy aspect of your uncontrolled snacking. Put it into practice immediately and refine it as necessary.

WORKSHEET

Use a Trick to Solve a Snacking Problem

Problem:

_____

_____

What I'll do:

_____

_____

_____

_____

_____

_____

Example:

Problem: Buying an ice-cream cone when I go to the dry-cleaners because I pass my favorite ice-cream shop

What I'll Do:

1. Change dry-cleaners, or
2. Take a different route to the dry-cleaners, or
3. Go to the dry-cleaners only in the morning before work, when the ice cream shop is closed (best solution).

9

Exercise: The Final Frontier

his chapter will teach you at least two new things about exercise. It is important to look at exercise in a new light especially if you do not have a workout program currently in place.

When I was a dieter, I would exercise whenever I went on a strict diet. My idea of exercise at that time was sit-ups, leg raises, and other slimnastic types of exertion. Aerobic exercise was something I rarely considered. Oh, occasionally I would try jogging, but because I was so out of shape and overweight, I would either become easily exhausted or would injure myself. It always meant that I would immediately quit out of frustration. Then, when I was off my strict diet, there seemed no point to exercising because my eating was back to its usual uncontrolled tendencies. To a degree, my thinking was not totally incorrect. After all, one can always easily exceed the calories burned in exercise by overeating.

In reality, that is not a good argument for not exercising. There is as much to be said for the mental discipline and benefits exercising provides, as for the physical results.

Most people who undertake a serious diet program will also begin some physical exercise, such as running, biking, swimming, or aerobics classes. Very few of these people will tell you they look forward to sweating and working hard for thirty to sixty minutes three to six times a week, although most will admit they feel better when they exercise. When their motivation wanes, however, they adhere less strictly to the diet. The person realizes that he is binge eating and that exercise cannot possibly compensate for it. At that point the person says, ''Something has to go! It doesn't make any sense to sweat my butt off and then keep breaking my diet.'' So, the exercise disappears along with the good eating habits, despite the fact that the person has admitted he feels better after exercising. His common sense also tells him that some positive effort is better than none.

But what if it worked another way? What if the person made a commitment to exercise five times per week, no matter what? He would have to set up a schedule whereby each week would begin on the same day. For example from Sunday to the following Saturday, five days of exercise must be completed, even if this means exercising five days in a row. This requires discipline! Which is exactly the point.

When the individual is eating in control and exercising regularly, everything is in balance. But when the eating becomes less controlled, you must force yourself to keep your other commitment to exercise, no matter what. If you continue to exercise five times per week for thirty to sixty minutes, you will eventually come to hate wasting this amount of time and will find some way to bring your eating back under control. Or at least your next attempt to control your eating will happen sooner.

In this way you will begin to establish what I call a *foundation*. Chapter 25 will discuss this term more extensively, but for now let's say it is the development of a set of behaviors and disciplines that are independent of eating, but that have a positive effect on your weight and your feeling of better health and well-being.

In order to control your weight permanently, exercise must become a part of your foundation. I have just described how exercise is generally related to the success or failure of a diet. Sometimes it is difficult to separate the two, but the two must remain independent. After all, you don't stop brushing your teeth just because your diet isn't going well, do you? The same principle must be applied to exercise. Now here's how to get with it.

As mentioned above, we generally think of two types of exercise. One is the slimnastic type (sit-ups, leg raises, and push-ups). The other is the aerobic type (running, jogging, biking, swimming, et cetera). The most important exercise is the aerobic type.

Aerobic exercise is more important because it burns fat and stimulates your metabolism, which you need. This form of exercise will help bring your eating behavior under control. Studies have repeatedly shown the importance of aerobic exercise in losing weight and maintaining the loss, by positively affecting the heart and circulatory system.

Once you accept the importance of aerobic exercise, find out what is aerobic for you. Aerobic fitness occurs when the person achieves an aerobic heart rate and maintains it for a particular amount of time. The activity must then be done a particular number of times per week for maximum benefit. Look at the chart below to determine your aerobic heart rate. Choose an activity to do at least three days per week that will help you achieve this heart rate for twenty minutes every time.

Aerobic conditioning is achieved when the heart is in the target range for at least twenty consecutive minutes three days per week. This will be your initial goal.

Aerobic Pulse Range

Age	Pulse	Age	Pulse
15–20	140–160	45–55	120–140
20–25	135–155	55–65	110–130
25–35	130–150	65–75	100–120
35–45	125–145	75–85	90–110

To count your pulse: When you stop exercising, quickly place the tips of your middle and index fingers lightly over one of the blood vessels in your neck located on either side of your Adam's apple. Another spot to check is the inside of your wrist just below the base of your thumb. Count your pulse for ten seconds and multiply by six. If your pulse is below the pulse target zone listed above, exercise a bit harder. If it is above the pulse target zone, exercise a little easier. If you are in the target zone, you're doing fine as long as you don't feel exhausted. There is no advantage to pushing too fast, too soon. Check your pulse at least once in the middle of each exercise routine.

If you are on blood pressure or other heart medication, this may slow your heart rate and you will not be able to achieve the target listed above. That's fine, as long as you feel slightly pushed when you exercise. If you are in any doubt about this, consult your physician.

It is important eventually to exercise at this target zone for at least twenty minutes, three times per week. In doing so you will reach the fat-burning potential of aerobic exercise. Your body will burn carbohydrates (stored in the body from starches, breads, and the like) before it burns fat. Since it is important to use up stored fat from the body, the longer the exercise, the more likely the body is to burn carbohydrate calories and then switch to fat calories. Also, you won't be eating while exercising, which is certainly desirable.

An incentive to exercise more often is both the extra calories burned each week and the way in which it affects your metabolism. With aerobic exercise, there is an increase in the amount of calories burned for up to twelve hours after the exercise ends. Therefore, the more often you exercise, the more you speed up your metabolism.

For these and many other reasons, you are advised to exercise at least five days a week for forty-five minutes each time and never less than thirty minutes. This is your ultimate goal and should be gradually worked toward depending on your current level of conditioning. Remember, the exercise must be continuous. You can not take two fifteen-minute walks and count that as aerobic exercise.

Now that you know how often to exercise, you may be wondering when to exercise. There are many opinions on this matter. There are two advantages to exercising first thing in the morning. The first is that the carbohydrates stored in the body burn more when the body has been fasting for the longest period of time in the day. That would be after awakening and before eating anything. Under these circumstances, the body is ready to switch to the fat-burning mode more quickly than at any other time during the day. The second reason for exercising first thing in the morning is that you get it out of the way. Many people will admit that whenever they leave something like exercising for later in the day, they encounter obstacles that prevent them from accomplishing their goal.

Now that I've probably persuaded you to exercise in the morning let me make some very good points in favor of exercising in the late afternoon or early evening when you first get out of work. Although almost everyone feels too exhausted to exercise after work, remember that exercise is an energizer. When you feel like taking a nap at two o'clock on a cloudy Sunday afternoon, the best thing you can do is take a forty-five minute brisk walk. Both the nap and the exercise will leave you feeling refreshed. It's just that the exercise will leave you with a greater sense of accomplishment.

Another advantage to exercising before dinner is that the exercise will cut down your appetite prior to the toughest meal of the day. Really! The first thing a stressed worker wants to do when he gets home is eat. The first thing he should do is put on aerobic shoes and go out walking. This will stop him from getting into snacking, then when he returns forty-five minutes later, if he drinks a large glass of water his cravings will be more in control. Remember how important this is, because, as I mentioned earlier, eating after 3:00 P.M. is usually the first step in letting our eating habits get out of control.

In answering the original question—when should I exercise?—try both. See what works best for you. Eventually, settle on a routine that includes exercise before dinner at least three days a week. Continue this pattern until your eating habits are under significantly better control.

Last, a brief explanation of various aerobic activities and their advantages:

Walking briskly. This is probably the best overall exercise. All you need is a good pair of shoes. Almost everyone can do this unless he or she has some significant physical impairment.

Jogging. It is now believed that there is no great advantage to jogging in favor of walking briskly. Also, there is more likelihood of a jogger injuring himself, which would then give him a legitimate excuse for not exercising for a while.

Biking. This can be either an indoor or an outdoor activity. Both provide a good workout as long as you avoid pedaling at too high an intensity at times and don't coast. Keep the seat extended so that each knee is only slightly bent when the leg is fully extended. That way, the knees are not unduly stressed.

Aerobic dancing. You can do this at gym/health club classes, by renting an aerobic videotape, or in many areas of the country by following aerobic exercise classes offered on TV. It is one of the best indoor exercises. It is also why I never let people who travel extensively stop exercising, since they can easily bring a headphone and cassette player and walk or do aerobic dancing to music. This also happens to be the perfect exercise for people who spend most of their time in the house with children, since it can be done at virtually any time with little preparation.

Swimming/pool jogging. I never mention swimming without immediately mentioning pool jogging because most people cannot swim continuously for forty-five minutes. Pool jogging, however, is walking and bouncing around in the water with the water at waist level. This is an excellent exercise for those who are physically impaired, because the water absorbs body weight and makes movement much easier. Recent studies show, however, that swimming may not be as likely to burn fat as is walking or biking.

If you still claim that you do not have time to exercise, consider the following two points. First, are you ready to state that you do not waste forty-five minutes on any given day? There are few people who are so organized that they still don't waste a good deal of time. If you become more organized, you will find time to exercise. And if you exercise, you probably will become more organized. It's a cycle, and one that will not entrap you. Second, if you state that you don't have time to exercise regularly, you must reevaluate your desire to lose weight and keep it off. Experts agree that it is virtually impossible to maintain weight loss if you do not have an aerobic exercise program.

So, get out there and do it. You'll feel 100 percent better. Your health will be improved. It will become a piece of your foundation to live with forever, just like brushing your teeth. Go for it!

Day 9 Assignment: If you have not already done so, choose one or more aerobic types of exercise (biking, jogging, dancing, walking) that interest you. Think about the next seven days and plan the minimum number of times you can do this activity during that week. Make the goal very easy to achieve! It is essential that at the end of the seven days you have done the amount of exercise you committed to without making excuses. Write the planned number of exercise times on the sheet provided at the end of this chapter and schedule the times for the workouts as if you were making appointments. Plan at least one of the exercise activities before a dinner meal.

WORKSHEET

Goal for Exercise for the Next Seven Days

DAY	ACTIVITY	AMOUNT OF TIME	TIME

Example:

Goal for exercise for the next seven days: I will exercise three days for no less than thirty minutes each time. At least one workout will be before dinner.

DAY	AMOUNT OF TIME	ACTIVITY	TIME
Tuesday	1 hour	Aerobic dancing	5:00 P.M.
Thursday	30 minutes	Stationary biking	7:00 A.M.
Saturday	40 minutes	Brisk walking	9:00 A.M.

10

Goal Orientation

*H*ow are you at goal setting? Most of us are pretty bad at it. We seldom write down goals that we wish to achieve, and, unfortunately, without putting goals on paper, they often remain ill-defined. More important, we never have that positive feeling of accomplishment when we don't know what our specific goals are.

In regard to eating, goal setting is a strong essential reinforcer of behavioral change. It has been shown repeatedly that positive reinforcement is far more effective in accomplishing change than is negative feedback.

The key words to goal setting in order to change eating habits are *small* and *achievable*. When initially learning this process, nothing is more important than being successful. When setting your first goals, choose ones that require minimal effort in order to get used to doing them routinely.

For example, when Diane got married four years ago she had only a slight weight problem, which normally she could control through working out and occasional dieting. Two years ago, Diane and Jim had a baby. Diane gained 45 pounds during her pregnancy but only lost 30 in the six months following delivery. Added to this fact, Diane now stays home with her daughter instead of going out to work. She gets bored often and finds her eating habits are seldom in control. In addition to the residual 15 pounds from pregnancy, Diane has gained another 20 pounds over the past eighteen months, so she now weighs almost as much as when she delivered Casey. Diane and Jim want to have another baby but Diane dreads what will happen to her weight and self-esteem if she gets pregnant now. She wants to lose weight, but nothing seems to work. She is extremely depressed over the way she looks and feels about herself.

Diane desperately needs to set some goals to deal with her eating habits and her life. If she's like most dieters, she has failed to lose weight because she tries to tackle the whole problem at once. Instead, she should try to break down her problem so that she can begin to feel a sense of accomplishment. As I stated previously, your first goals should require minimal effort to ensure success. For example; Diane has only minimal problems with snacking between lunch and dinner. This is primarily because she takes advantage of Casey's naptime to do some correspondence for Jim's business, which keeps her hands occupied. Therefore, her first goal should be to do Jim's correspondence at least three days a week, during which time she will not eat. Since she already does this two days a week, adding one day will not be hard to accomplish.

Diane feels her toughest problems begin when she puts the leftover food away after dinner. Jim has offered to do this for Diane so that when she does the dishes, she will not see any tempting food left on the plates.

If she continues to focus her energies on these types of behavioral changes, she will begin to lose weight just by solving her situational problems. Realistically, though, as she begins to see the slightest success in her weight as a result of her behavioral changes, she will undertake a diet as well. This is fine as long as the focus remains balanced between behavior, diet, and exercise.

Now let's look at the typical, overweight business executive. Weight problems are very difficult for all of us to deal with, but somehow they are even more exasperating to the executive. Why? Because he is a very successful, driven, and usually goal-oriented person who sees his weight problem as his Achilles' heel. It's a problem most can't solve. They diet, they are successful, and then in a very short time the problem returns. It virtually drives them crazy.

There are a couple of things that may help the executive and a few that may hinder him. On a positive note, these people are generally, as mentioned, "driven"—meaning that they are highly motivated and put a great deal of energy into what they do. Since controlling what one eats is basically a lifelong process, it will never come naturally and it will always require motivation. You probably will never find that you are "cured." The creative side of the executive helps here also in that a long-term task requires new solutions from time to time, and this is a concept with which he is usually familiar.

Another advantage the typical executive has is that he is most likely goal oriented, and written-goal oriented at that! He already knows how to break down goals into their various components. Such goal orientation can be a problem if the executive is accustomed to delegating tasks to others in order to accomplish his goals, for he will not be accustomed to doing the tasks himself. Obviously this will create problems. Let's look at a few.

If an individual spends more time worrying about his business affairs than about himself, he will need to learn new behaviors to deal with his habits. But taking time for himself will not come easily. In addition, if he is the type of executive who delegates tasks to others, he may try to delegate the responsibility for his eating habits to co-workers or other people in his life. For example, he may blame his spouse for bringing food into the house without first trying to work out an agreement as to what the problem foods are and how to avoid them.

Josh is a thirty-two-year-old executive with a large computer technology firm. He's been out of school for ten years and recently received a promotion that assures he will be on the fast track to top management. He will be traveling about 30 percent of the time, which is a bit more than he does currently. He also entertains clients frequently at business dinners.

Josh has been married for six years and has a two-year-old son. His wife, Dana, does not work now and they are considering baby number two. Josh never had a weight problem in childhood or adolescence. He put on 10 extra pounds in college but then lost it by jogging and drinking less beer.

Currently, Josh's weight is 15 pounds above his low maintenance weight in college. He doesn't look fat, but he feels more comfortable at the lower weight. At his most recent company physical, the doctor noted a high cholesterol count and told Josh to lower the fat in his diet and to exercise. Josh hasn't felt he has had the time to exercise since he got married.

The main problems in Josh's health and diet picture are no exercise, eating appetizers in restaurants (he loves cheese sticks), too much alcohol intake (when entertaining he also snacks on peanuts etc.), eating too late at night, and skipping meals (always breakfast and often lunch).

What would you work on first if you were Josh? One of the best things would be to return to jogging or some other exercise program. He should make a written goal of what he wants to do, what time of the day he wants to do it, and how often he is willing to do it initially. Since this is an area in which he was successful before and it had a positive effect on his weight at that time, he already has a positive association with which to connect. Another incentive for Josh to exercise is the positive effect it will have on his cholesterol when combined with a low-fat diet. Last, when anyone makes a commitment to exercise, he is more likely to take all kinds of positive steps in his life.

For example, diet improves, stress is managed better, and the use of nonprescription medication decreases. The main caution for Josh regarding exercise is that he must guard against trying to do too much too soon. It is common for executives to start out exercising every day, then burn out or injure themselves, and then not exercise again for a long time. It is important to start out slowly, keep up the variety, and make the goals achievable.

Next, Josh should write a list of goals concerning the other areas that are small and achievable:

1. Limit appetizers in restaurants to once a week for a high-fat appetizer, once a week for a healthy appetizer.

2. Limit alcohol to one mixed drink or one glass of wine per night during the week, and one of each or two of one on the weekend. Limit nibbles to pretzels during the week and potato chips on only one weekend day.

3. When working late at the office, go to the cafeteria and buy a big salad to bring back to his desk, in the hope that he will eat lighter when he gets home.

4. Don't change skipping lunch on occasion, but try to drink a glass of milk for breakfast each morning.

Now, none of these changes represents perfect eating behavior, nor are they the only steps to be taken. They are, however, very positive steps toward improving control over eating habits. More important, to Josh, they are changes he can achieve and live with.

Such goals can be a big boost in helping you to feel in control of all aspects of your life. Don't take on too much at once, or you will lose sight of your overall goal. Rewarding yourself when a goal is accomplished is the missing piece of the equation, and that will be discussed in chapter 22. Till then write down your goals and achieve them!

Day 10 Assignment: Before you attempt to set new goals, think about some of the changes you have already made, but not written down. Now, write them down as part of your written goals if you have been accomplishing them consistently. The most important thing about goals initially is that you can accomplish them and that you feel good about accomplishing them. After you have done this, add one goal that you have not yet been accomplishing consistently, but think you now can.

WORKSHEET

Behaviors I've Been Accomplishing but Not Previously Written

1. _____

2. _____

3. _____
4. _____

Behaviors I've Yet to Accomplish Consistently but Will Now

1. _____
2. _____
3. _____

Examples:

Behaviors I've Been Accomplishing but Not Previously Written

1. I have been eating a small carton of yogurt every afternoon instead of candy.

2. I have been eating breakfast at least three days a week.

3. I have not bought ice cream for the house.

4. I have not used regular salad dressing on my salad.

Behaviors I've Yet to Accomplish Consistently but Will Now

1. I will weigh my entree before putting it on my plate.

2. I will use only a fat substitute on my baked potato and avoid butter, margarine, and sour cream each time with a

margin of twice a month for the "real stuff" if I want them.

3. I will eat breakfast at least five days a week.

_____

11

In Search of Fat

I hope you're reading this book in sequence, because this, one of the most important chapters, absolutely must be read before chapter 12, "The Basic Forever Eating Plan."

Also, as ironic as it may sound, this chapter has less to do with the how-to's of changing your eating habits than does any other chapter. It does, however, provide the basis for the direction your behavioral change will take.

If you ask most people what are the greatest problems in their eating habits, they will frequently say, "sweets"; this is the food they lose control of most frequently. But if you ask them what it is about the sweets that attracts them, they will say they crave sugar. However, if you tell them to have a gumdrop the next time they have a sweets craving, the odds are they will reply that's not what they really want. That's because it is the **fat** in sweets that we really crave, and it's far more detrimental to our diet and weight than is sugar.

A dieter knows where the sugar is in his diet. He knows if he puts sugar in his coffee or tea, if he drinks regular sodas, and which sweets he eats that have sugar in them, although you sometimes have to remind dieters that ice cream is a sweet too, since we often categorize it by itself. But ask the person where the fat is in his diet and he will have a hard time. He will tell you that he doesn't eat fried foods, always takes the skin off the chicken, and may not even put sour cream on his baked potatoes anymore. Therefore, he thinks he is consuming a low-fat diet. In most cases, he still doesn't have a clue as to how much fat is in his diet.

The typical American diet derives 38 to 45 percent of its calories from fat. The American Dietetic Association and other health organizations recommend that less than 30 percent of one's calories come from fat. The question you may have at this point is: Why is fat so important? This is an excellent question if you have always been a calorie watcher in the past.

Experts once thought that calories alone were the key factor in weight loss. It was a simple equation: When the body burned 3,500 excess calories, the person lost 1 pound. We always knew that fat has more calories by weight:

Fat	1 gram	9 calories
Alcohol	1 gram	6 calories

| Protein | I gram | 4 calories |
| Carbohydrate | I gram | 4 calories |

Note: A gram is 1/454 of a pound.

These measurements were taken into account when calculating the caloric content of foods. In other words, it was thought that as long as a person cut down on his calories, to 1,000 a day for example, he would lose weight even if he ate a high-fat diet. If he squeezed a candy bar into his 1,000-calorie plan, it did not affect his weight loss any more than if he didn't cheat at all and ate a "healthful" 1,000 calories. Of course, there would be less food in a high-fat diet, due to the caloric density of high-fat foods. For example, the following foods each contain the same number of calories but differ in quantity and filling ability:

3 cups cauliflower
1/3 cup pasta
3 Hershey's Kisses

All contain about 75 calories. The difference is that the cauliflower is more filling because it provides bulk and water. As there is virtually no fat, the quantity is generous.

Now we know that it is not just a matter of the quantity of calories consumed but of the type of calories. And it is making a big difference in how people diet.

Recent studies tell us that fat turns to fat more easily. That makes sense, doesn't it? The theory is based on the observation that foods high in carbohydrate (bread, pasta, potatoes, rice, cereal, fruit, et cetera) burn better than fatty foods. That extra burning potential can actually account for additional calories used in the digestion process. This is the opposite of the fat-burning process, which seems to slow down the body's digestion and metabolism and therefore turns the fat more easily into fat.

This explanation makes it apparent why some people who have cut their calories significantly still haven't lost much weight. The fat in their diets is most likely too high. This is often the case because the diet frequently adopted is that of the 1970s—that is, a high-protein diet—which increases the intake of meats, eggs, cheeses, and other high-fat foods.

Now that you know that fat is worse than other components of a diet, let's identify the sources of fat in your diet:

Animal products
Added fats
Fats in commercial products

Each will be discussed separately and in depth. It is vital to learn to search for the fat in your diet.

The largest contributor of fat in the diet is animal products and by-products. The reason for identifying the foods as animal, rather than as meat, is that people generally assume that meat refers only to red meat. Since we don't want to be that limited, I'll use the term *animal products*.

There are a few reasons why animal products are the

main source of dietary fat. First, animal products derive as much as 80 percent or more of their calories from fat. This means that just eating a small portion yields many fat calories. Second, we are entrée oriented. Since the Depression of the 1930s, putting a decent piece of meat on the plate has been a sign of good providership. Although the plate may contain a starch and a vegetable, the entrée (the meat) is the focal point. It also takes up the largest part of the plate. Because of this, think about how off-balanced a plate would look if the starch and vegetable were huge and the entrée much smaller. It would make your brain unhappy, and your brain has the ability to make your stomach very unhappy. Ultimately, that leads to a lot of unplanned snacking.

Are all animal products culprits? No, not all of them contribute high amounts of fat. What about the importance of animal products in contributing protein to the diet? This is important, but not as much as you may think. (Chapter 15 deals extensively with protein.)

The following information will give you an idea of the fat composition of many animal products. It also shows how you can obtain plenty of protein without consuming plenty of fat.

Group 1 derives more fat calories than protein per ounce. *Cheeses*: most of them; *fatty meats*: brisket, ribs, and those with heavy marbling; *processed meats*: bologna, frank-furters, bacon, sausage, duck, goose, et cetera.

Group 2 is still very fatty. *Reduced-fat cheeses* (except cottage cheese), part-skimmed mozzarella, et cetera; *meats with medium marbling*: steaks, chops, roasts, poultry consumed with the skin; *fatty fish*: salmon (fresh, canned fish packed in oil); *eggs: regular cottage cheese*.

Group 3 starts to hit a more acceptable balance between fat and protein. *Poultry consumed without the skin; 95–97 percent fat-free luncheon meats; lean red meats*; flank steak, round steak, tenderloin, lean pork chops, veal scaloppini.

Group 4 animal products are so lean that the fat content barely counts. *turkey breast and other 97–99 percent fat-free luncheon meats; 1 percent cottage cheese; skim milk; nonfat yogurt; egg whites; very lean fish*: sole, flounder, cod, and shellfish,

The above will help you understand where an animal product falls in terms of fat content. The following rules of thumb will enable you to make quick decisions regarding their inclusion in your diet.

1. **Avoid cheeses as much as possible except for 1 percent cottage cheese.** An ounce of turkey breast has 1 gram of fat. An ounce of part-skim mozzarella has 5 grams of fat—that's 500 percent more, and you cannot often afford that.
2. **Try to have at least one selection daily from Group 4 for either lunch or dinner.**
3. **Choose your breakfast protein from Group 4 at least six days a week.**

Taking these suggestions and remembering sources of fat in animal products will get you to look at animal products in a whole new light. Then you're on your way!

Fats added to foods include: butter, margarine, oils, salad dressing, peanut butter, cream cheese, sour cream, and mayonnaise. Don't confuse the term *no-cholesterol* with *no-* or *low-fat*. **Fat is fat!** The cholesterol content has nothing to do with the amount of fat in a product. *Added fat should be avoided as much as possible*. The theory that we need added fat in the diet for lubrication is not valid, unless the person is a vegetarian.

There are three questions that you should ask yourself when considering adding a fat to food. The first is, "Is there a product I can use that does not contain fat?" The answer to this is often *yes*. In place of butter or margarine, peanut butter or cream cheese, use low-sugar jam. In place of oil in cooking, use no-stick spray or cook with wine. In place of sour cream use nonfat yogurt. In place of regular salad dressing, use fat-free salad dressing.

When the answer to the first question has yielded a *no*, the second question to ask yourself is, "Is there a low-fat item I can substitute?" In place of mayonnaise, use light mayonnaise. In place of margarine, use a small amount of reduced-calorie margarine. In place of sour cream, use a small amount of light sour cream. In place of regular salad dressing, use a small amount of low-fat salad dressing.

When the answers to the first two questions are still *no* (as when you are in a restaurant), eat the item plain, if possible. If you can't bear the thought of that, use the real thing but only very little of it. For example, make sure to order salad dressing on the side.

The last category is fat in commercial products. This

can be a tricky area, particularly if you consume a lot of convenience foods. I recommend that fat in the diet should be 30 percent or less of the total calories, which means each food you consume should derive less than thirty percent of its calories from fat. To calculate the percentage of calories from fat in a product:

> **Multiply the grams of fat by 9.**
> **Divide that number by the total number of calories.**
> **Multiply that number by 100 to get the percent.**
> **Choose those foods which derive 30 percent or less of their calories from fat.**

For example:

> A frozen diet dinner has 290 calories and 13 grams of fat:
> 13 × 9 = 117 calories from fat
> 117 divided by 290 = .40 × 100 = 40 percent of calories from fat

There are some simple rules to use in evaluating the fat content of foods. These rules don't require taking a calculator to the grocery store. When looking at the nutritional analysis on the label, first make sure you understand what a serving is, since nutritional analyses are always based on a per-serving portion. When looking at the label on an item that will be a complete meal, such as a frozen dinner, 10 or fewer grams of fat is a good rule of thumb. When looking at an individual item, 3 or fewer grams of fat is the rule, as long as you stick with consuming only a single portion.

The following chart gives approximations of the fat content of various foods. Use it as a guide in making decisions. It is by no means a complete analysis of all foods available for consumption, but it is a good basic guideline.

Remember, the rule of thumb is that there should be no greater than 3 grams of fat in a single serving of a product. There should be no greater than 3 grams of fat per ounce. And allow no more than 10 grams of fat in a complete-meal item.

FOOD PRODUCT	SERVING SIZE	GRAMS OF FAT
DAIRY		
Cheese, most hard	1 ounce	6–10
Cheese, cream	2 tablespoons	10
Cheese, Alpine Lace	1 ounce	8
Cheese, cottage	½ cup	5
Cheese, cottage 1%	½ cup	2
Cheese, Lite Line	1 ounce	2
Whipped cream	1 tablespoon	6
Half and half	2 tablespoons	4
Milk, whole	8 ounces	8

FOOD PRODUCT	SERVING SIZE	GRAMS OF FAT
DAIRY		
Milk, 2%	8 ounces	5
Milk, skim	8 ounces	*
Eggnog	8 ounces	20
Yogurt, nonfat	8 ounces	*
Yogurt, low fat	8 ounces	4
Pudding, whole milk	½ cup	4
Ice cream, premium	½ cup	12
Ice milk	½ cup	5
Sour cream	2 tablespoons	5
MEATS		
Spare ribs	3 ounces	26
Brisket	3 ounces	15
Ground beef, 27% fat	3 ounces	17
Ground beef, 18% fat	3 ounces	14
Beef, medium marbleing	3 ounces	9–13
Tenderloin	3 ounces	4
Lamb, trimmed	3 ounces	8–12
Pork chop	3 ounces	13
Ham shank	3 ounces	12
Sausage, brown and serve	3 ounces	32
Bacon	3 slices	9

FOOD PRODUCT	SERVING SIZE	GRAMS OF FAT
POULTRY		
Chicken with skin	3 ounces	13
Chicken, white no skin	3 ounces	4
Chicken, dark, no skin	3 ounces	6
Turkey, white, no skin	3 ounces	4
Turkey franks	3 ounces	16
Turkey breast, deli	3 ounces	3
Turkey sausage	3 ounces	16
Turkey, ground	3 ounces	9
Duck, flesh and skin	3 ounces	24
FISH		
White: flounder, scrod, grouper, halibut, etc.	3 ounces	3–6
Dark: tuna, salmon, mackerel	3 ounces	14
Shellfish	3 ounces	3–6
EGGS		
Whole	1 large	6
White only	1 large	0
Yolk only	1 large	6
Eggbeaters	¼ cup	0

FOOD PRODUCT	SERVING SIZE	GRAMS OF FAT
CRACKERS		
Ritz	5	5
Saltines	5	2
Triscuits	5	4
Krispen	5	*
Melba Toast	5	1
FATS		
Oil, any brand	1 tablespoon	14
Butter/margarine	1 tablespoon	14
Butter Buds	1 tablespoon	0
Salad dressing, regular	1 tablespoon	6–9
Mayonnaise	1 tablespoon	11
Diet mayo	1 tablespoon	5
Cream cheese	2 tablespoons	10
Peanut butter	2 tablespoons	14
STARCHES		
Potato, pasta, rice, bread, cereal (most)	½ cup	2
VEGETABLES		
All	½ cup	2

FOOD PRODUCT	SERVING SIZE	GRAMS OF FAT
FRUITS		
All	medium or ½ cup	0
MISCELLANEOUS		
Nuts	1 ounce	12–16
Coconut	1 ounce	12
Seeds	1 ounce	16–20
Avocado	1 medium	30

*Less than 1 gram of fat.

Day 11 Assignment: Using the above table of fat content of various foods, compare some of your early food records and calculate the grams of fat contained in your diet. Notice how even though you were trying to limit the quantity, the fat intake was still higher than recommended.

WORKSHEET

Food Diary

FOOD	TIME OF DAY	PLACE	WITH WHOM	FAT GRAMS
8 ounces skim milk	8:30 A.M.	kitchen	alone	0
¾ cup cornflakes				2

SNACK ATTACK

Food	Time of Day	Place	With Whom	Fat Grams
banana				0
coffee with 1 teaspoon sugar				0
ham sandwich	1:00 P.M.			12
potato chips—1 ½ oz bag		deli	co-worker	10
soda—12 ounces				0
candy bar—2 oz	4:00	desk	alone	9
handful of nuts	5:30	kitchen	alone	14
½ chicken breast	6:30	table	spouse	9
1 cup mashed potatoes				5
small ear of corn				0
margarine—2 tablespoons				10
salad—2 tablespoons dressing				14
Iced tea—2 teaspoons sugar				0
1 8 oz cup of ice cream	8:00	TV room	spouse	16
			Total Fat Grams	101

12

The Basic Forever Eating Plan

Day 12 Assignment: This chapter and chapter 13 are inseparable, as the Basic Forever Eating Plan includes a snacking plan. In chapter 13, you will see the calorie-controlled meal plans for 1,000, 1,200, and 1,500 calories. For now, write an eating plan for a day based on the guidelines in this chapter. Remember to keep your preferences included in the plan. It is important to like what you eat, otherwise this is not a "forever plan" but just another diet. In the next chapter, see how your plan compares to the actual calorie-controlled meal plans.

During this entire chapter, do not ever forget why the word *forever* is in the title. There is no point in making changes in your eating habits unless you can live with them the majority of the time. Don't expect perfection all the time, but do strive to feel in control.

When a livable eating plan is adopted, there is no food that can never be eaten. The person just learns to eat more of the best and less of the rest. When on an unlivable diet, the dieter longs for forbidden food, and when not adhering to the diet, he is frequently bingeing. This usually means that when the dieter "cheats" with a cookie, for example, he then thinks he may as well get everything he has been craving out of his system.

Furthermore, the unlivable diet can be successful only once. Liquid diets are the perfect example of this. Drinking five milkshakes a day and consuming no food is hardly livable, especially if the dieter is successful in losing weight but then regains it. It becomes much more difficult to adhere to the liquids-only plan after the first time.

It is far better to plan and write a meal plan you can live with forever. There are some essential structural basics in writing one, and once these have been taken into account, filling in the food items is easy. If you can learn to think in terms of this structure, you will place less emphasis on the actual foods. This will mitigate your emotional resistance to making changes in your eating habits.

The first part of the structure is fat. For reasons cited in the preceding chapter, the Forever Eating Plan must be low in fat.

Next, remember not to fall victim to the 10/90 rule. If you don't remember this, review chapter 6. The meal plan must be written such that you consume at least 50 percent of your calories by 3:00 P.M., or whatever the midpoint of your day is. Additionally, two meals and two snacks should be planned before the day's midpoint. This will allow for optimum metabolism and the elimination of physical hunger.

There should not be a stretch longer than three hours between meals or snacks except from bedtime to awakening. This too keeps the individual from getting hungry and prevents slowing of the metabolism.

Those are the basic rules. Now let's look at actually writing the plan. We start with the most important meal of the day—breakfast.

Breakfast is essential for many reasons, the most important of which is that when it is not eaten, the body may perceive a state of starvation and slow its metabolism in response. That's the last thing you want to happen. Eating breakfast will also help you keep within the 50/50 rule. You will find it difficult to eat 50 percent of your calories before 3:00 P.M. if you skip breakfast.

Eating breakfast is also essential in helping control eating after dinner. Surprising, but true. What you eat in the morning affects how satiated you are at the end of the day. If you think that breakfast makes you hungrier, that you are actually better off on the days when you go as long as possible without eating—think again. What happens once you start eating? Most times you lose control. This meal plan will make sure you are not hungrier because you ate breakfast.

Breakfast must include lean and digestible protein. The best choices are:

8 ounces skim milk	8 ounces nonfat yogurt
1 egg	2 egg whites
1 ounce low-fat ham	⅓ cup 1% cottage cheese

Protein is digested more slowly than carbohydrate and therefore it sticks with you longer. Breakfast must also include a carbohydrate; bread and/or cereal are the usual choices (quantities will be given in the specific meal plans at the end of this chapter).

Snacks will be discussed in the following chapter, but you will find them written into the meal plan here. That brings us to lunch. There are many reasons why people make poor choices at lunch: they can't take time away from work, or it may not be possible for them to bring a home-packed lunch. However, this essential meal lends itself to a variety of options.

The most important aspect of eating lunch is to do it without distraction. Remember not to eat at your desk while working, for it will deprive you of the mental and therefore physical satisfaction of eating.

Lunch, like breakfast, must include protein. Again, this meal must stimulate your metabolism in order to sustain you until your next snack. By doing this you are laying a foundation that will prevent your appetite from getting out of control later on. Eating a fruit salad for lunch will not provide you with adequate staying power, because it doesn't have enough protein. Frozen yogurt doesn't have enough either, for despite the fact that it contains some milk, the product is almost exclusively made up of carbohydrates. The following are examples of luncheon foods that provide protein. (Quantities will be discussed in detail in the individual meal plans.)

95–99% fat-free luncheon meats	Nonfat yogurt
Water-packed tuna	1% cottage cheese
Imitation crab meat	Water-packed salmon
Leftover chicken breast or turkey	
Frozen dinner with 10 grams of fat or less	
One egg or 2 egg whites	

Last, we move on to dinner, the *least* important meal of the day. Yet it is the one meal we seem never to miss. Since our metabolisms are slower at night, our bodies have a harder time digesting this meal.

This is further complicated when we snack after dinner, because we go to sleep on those extra calories. When I advise someone to cut his dinner portion in half, he generally exclaims that this will cause him to snack all night. But he already snacks at night, even after eating a heavy dinner! Cutting the dinner portion will help reduce the overall caloric intake. Remember that we nibble for a variety of behavioral reasons that have little to do with true hunger or what we consume at dinner.

Unlike breakfast and lunch, dinner does not need to sustain your appetite, because you are going to bed soon and probably will not have to do any more work requiring a lot of energy. In addition, you will eat two more snacks before bedtime. Therefore, there is no need to eat protein at dinner. The closer you are to being a vegetarian at this meal, the easier it will be to control your appetite permanently. There are numerous easy and delicious ways to accomplish this.

Since you will pretty much continue to eat dinner seven nights a week, you must learn to live by the **2-2-2-1 rule**. This rule will help you keep a running tally on how your dinners fit in with your overall meal plan. It also keeps you focused on the structure of the plan rather than on what you actually eat.

2 nights a Week, the Dinner Will Be VEGETARIAN

This means that animal products and most animal by-products will be avoided. Remember that by eliminating this from dinner twice every week you will help reduce your fat intake significantly. Vegetarian meals consist of: meatless spaghetti; beans and rice; a baked potato and vegetables; 1% cottage cheese and fruit; vegetable soup and a roll; cereal and skim milk. Portions will be specified in the written meal plans.

2 dinners Will Be Lean Fish or Shellfish

I frequently hear from my clients, "I eat a lot of fish and chicken." The truth is, they eat a lot of chicken. They don't eat much fish. The reasons for this vary from not knowing how to cook it, to the fact that another member of the family doesn't like fish. It is important, however, to eat more fish and shellfish since it is usually significantly leaner than chicken. Lean fish include flounder, sole, grouper, cod, scrod, and other fish that appears white when raw. This does not include salmon, mackerel, sardines, or tuna, which are more like chicken in their fat content. The reason most often cited for avoiding shellfish is its cholesterol content. This is a factor only with shrimp and lobster, and even then it is not that significant a problem. (More about this in chapter 14.)

2 Nights a Week—Stir-Fry Without Oil

The goal at dinner is to keep the portion of chicken, turkey, or beef to a maximum of 3 ounces. This amounts to the size of a deck of cards. That sight can be pretty depressing to many meat eaters, so stir-frying is their answer. Consider the following.

You and your spouse are going to have filet mignon for dinner. They seemed reasonably small portions but now that you look at the package, you find that they are actually 8 ounces each! In order to eat 3 ounces or less, cook just one steak (we'll assume 2 ounces of shrinkage) and freeze the other portion. After cooking the steak, divide it into two equal portions and serve it with rice and vegetable(s). The once-adequate filet now looks like a morsel of meat on the plate. Your spouse, expecting the usual portion, threatens to leave you if you ever do this again.

However, if you sliced that same filet into a hundred strips, then stir-fried it with nonstick spray, a dash of wine, and tons of vegetables, and served it over rice, the meal would have great eye appeal and rarely would anyone complain that there wasn't enough meat. You might even have leftovers!

This is why stir-frying without oil is an excellent way of preparing animal products. Try to make only one of the stir-fry dinners consist of beef, pork, or veal. The other stir-fry meal can be either skinless chicken breast or skinless turkey breast.

1 Night a Week—Have Any Entrée You Want

Just be reasonable on the portion. This will allow you to enjoy your old favorites.

Those are the basic guidelines of the meal plan. The calorie plans presented later are inclusive of the above structure. The suggestions are interchangeable within a specific meal—i.e., any breakfast can be selected and combined with any lunch. But you must remember to keep the 2-2-2-1 rule.

Write your own meal plan on the worksheet that follows. Suggestions for snacks will be given in the next chapter. After reading them, you can fill in your snack plans.

WORKSHEET

Meal Plan

BREAKFAST

SNACK

LUNCH

SNACK

DINNER

SNACK

SNACK

Example:

Breakfast
1 egg
1 piece toast
1 teaspoon margarine
1 teaspoon jelly
Coffee with 1 teaspoon sugar

SNACK:
1 piece of fruit

LUNCH
½ can (6½ ounce can) water-packed tuna
2 pieces bread
2 teaspoons low-calorie mayonnaise
Lettuce
Apple
Iced tea with sweetener

SNACK
5 ounces nonfat frozen yogurt

DINNER
5 ounces shrimp

Medium baked potato

2 tablespoons low-fat sour cream

1 cup broccoli

Salad with 2 tablespoons nonfat dressing

SNACK
½ cup cereal

½ cup 1% milk

SNACK
½ cup strawberries

13

Snacking: It's All in the Plan

You've read what adopting new eating habits involves. Because there are plenty of opportunities for snacking, let's now get into the real nuts and bolts of how to control uncontrolled nibbling once a solid foundation is laid.

There are various ways to deal with uncontrolled snacking, but one of the best is to plan for it. In other words, know that there is a distinct possibility that you may have a problem. I had a client who told me she was having a small problem with miniature Almond Joy bars. She was eating five every night. This is certainly not even close to the damage nibblers usually do, but it was still troublesome. I told her I was sure that we could solve the problem, but that she would have to do it my way. Desperately, she agreed.

The first step was to write a snacking plan. First, attempt

to duplicate your usual behavior for one day. My client's snack plan read as follows

```
┌─────────────────────────────────────────┐
│                                         │
│            Night Snack Plan             │
│                                         │
│     7 P.M.          Almond Joy          │
│     8 P.M.          Almond Joy          │
│     9 P.M.          Almond Joy          │
│    10 P.M.          Almond Joy          │
│    11 P.M.          Almond Joy          │
│                                         │
└─────────────────────────────────────────┘
```

Of course, despite our agreement, my client did not want to continue her behavior for even one more day. What she wanted me to do was to make her stop eating the candy completely. But I assured her that changes made in an overnight fashion rarely last. We have seen why the cold-turkey approach to eating rarely works.

But, if my client replaced one Almond Joy bar with an alternate snack every other night, she would ultimately have to decide whether to eat one Almond Joy each night or phase them out completely. I told her to make the substitute snack appropriate: diet gelatin, a piece of low-calorie bread with jam, or air-popped popcorn.

The decision of whether or not to continue eating one Almond Joy bar is an important one. The ultimate goal here is to control what foods you eat. At the same time, a person must realize that control may never be possible with every food. Such danger foods must be identified and specific decisions made as to how to deal with them. The following should help you in this process.

Control Versus Abstinence

It is better to control than to abstain, unless you blow it. Then you'll wish you had abstained. That probably doesn't make sense upon first reading, but its essence will soon be clear.

When I finally began to get my eating habits under control, I lost 35 pounds and for once, I kept it off. During this time I faced many challenges, among them an array of goodies every Friday morning at the office. There were always either doughnuts, bagels, muffins, or danish pastries. At first I abstained from all of them because I wasn't ready to exhibit any level of control. But after a time I would take a small predecided amount and then no more. This felt even better than avoiding the food completely, because I controlled it. This worked for a long time, until someone brought in my absolute favorite dessert. I took my predetermined piece, then another, then another, et cetera. In other words, I blew it!

For all the times that I controlled my eating, I don't remember any one time specifically. However, I remember almost every detail about that one bad experience. We always focus more on our downfalls than our successes.

Control makes us feel wonderfully powerful. Abstinence, on the other hand, implies that we have no control and therefore must abstain. It is frustrating to know that an inanimate object like food controls us instead of vice versa. The equivalent is looking at a pencil sharpener and feeling it controls our behavior. Whenever possible, control should be exercised to enhance our mental power. However, as shown by the example above, if you doubt your ability to control, it is better to abstain.

If snacks are planned you will feel in control of your nibbling. You cannot anticipate every occasion, but you can plan for several snacks. Generally I recommend that snacks range from 50 to 75 calories. There is an allowance in each meal plan for a midmorning snack, a midafternoon snack, and two evening snacks. Therefore, the selections are the same for snack choices regardless of the calorie limit. The other criterion for snacks is that they contain no greater than 2 grams of fat. The following snacks meet the criteria of 50 to 75 calories and no greater than 2 grams of fat.

1 medium piece fresh fruit
1 5-ounce cup frozen nonfat yogurt (15 calories or fewer per ounce)
1 4-ounce cup nonfat regular yogurt (50-calorie variety)
1 Alba Milkshake made with water
1 slice 40-calorie bread, 1 slice turkey breast, a spread of mustard, lettuce and tomato
1 slice 40-calorie bread and 1 teaspoon low-sugar jam
3 Wasa-type crackers and 1 teaspoon low-sugar jam and 1 tablespoon 1% cottage cheese
2 Weight Watchers' Chocolate Mousse Bars
2 sugar-free Fudgsicles

3 cups air-popped popcorn
1 cup sugar-free hot cocoa
½ medium baked potato
5 pieces of Melba Toast
2 cups green beans

As you can see, there are many snacks that meet the criteria. Variety is an important consideration and it has been provided here. Lack of variety is frequently the reason why fad diets fail. It should be noted, however, that some people can tolerate a great deal of repetition without getting bored with their meal plans. You must decide, in a non-emotional way, when you are ready to do so. I encourage you to keep a lot of variety in your meal plan until you begin to feel in control of your eating habits. Plan snacks based on your preferences, but keep up the variety.

Calorie Controlled Meal Plans

Try to lose weight on the maximum amount of calories that your body will allow. Doing so will make maintenance of that weight loss much easier. It is also important that you don't cut your calories below 1,000 daily. If you claim that you can't lose weight on so many calories, stick with it and give your metabolism a chance to adjust.

The following guidelines work for most people.

Choose 1,500 calories daily if you are a male over 5'7"
Choose 1,200 calories daily if you are a male 5'7" or
    under

Choose 1,200 calories daily if you are a female over 5′5″

Choose 1,000 calories daily if you are a female 5′5″ or under, or if you have lost and regained weight numerous times before

The calorie levels that follow are approximations. Close to the official calorie levels reported, they are averages based on your selections within the meals and snacks.

Beverages, except milk, are not listed but are permissible as long as they contain fewer than 10 calories per serving. That means that coffee, tea, decaffeinated beverages, diet soda, and sparkling waters without sugar are permissible. That also means juices are not allowed. Juices are among the most wasted sources of calories, since they don't really fill you up and the nutrients they provide can be found elsewhere. Milk should be consumed only where it is listed on the meal plan.

A medium serving of fruit should be approximately the size of a tennis ball. The exceptions to this are as follows.

Berries	½ cup
Banana	½ medium
Grapes	15 medium
Cherries	10 medium
Mango	½ medium
Canned fruit, water packed	½ cup

In general, try to avoid canned fruit and dried fruit. Canned fruit lacks the quantity of fiber that fresh fruit contains. Dried fruit lacks the water content that fresh fruit provides and therefore the portion is so small that it rarely seems worth eating.

1,500 Calories

BREAKFAST
8 ounces skim or 1% milk
¾ cup cereal, cold or cooked
1 slice toast or 2 slices 40-calorie toast
2 teaspoons low-sugar jam
1 serving fresh fruit

OR
1 egg and the white of 1 additional egg
or 3 egg whites done in nonstick spray
2-ounce bagel (small) *or* 2 slices toast
or English muffin
1 serving fresh fruit

OR
⅓ cup 1% cottage cheese *or* 1 ounce 95% fat-free ham
2-ounce bagel *or* 2 slices toast *or* English muffin
1 serving fresh fruit

OR

8 ounces nonfat yogurt (100 calories)
2-ounce bagel *or* 2 slices toast *or* English muffin
1 serving fresh fruit

OR

French toast:
4 slices 40-calorie toast *or* 2 regular toast soaked in egg whites and skim milk and fried in butter-flavored nonstick spray
2 tablespoons low-calorie syrup
8 ounces skim *or* 1% milk

MIDMORNING SNACK

1 medium piece fresh fruit
OR   1 4-ounce cup nonfat regular yogurt (50-calorie variety)
OR   1 Alba Milkshake made with water
OR   1 slice 40-calorie bread and 1 teaspoon low-sugar jam
OR   3 Wasa-type crackers and 1 teaspoon low-sugar jam and 1 tablespoon 1% cottage cheese

LUNCH

3 ounces 95–99% fat-free luncheon meat
2 slices regular bread *or* 4 slices 40-calorie bread
Lettuce and tomato
1 tablespoon light mayonnaise
1 serving fresh fruit

OR

3 ounces water-packed tuna, salmon, *or* sardines
Large salad with raw vegetables
2 slices regular bread *or* 4 slices 40-calorie bread
or 10 Wasa crackers *or* 2 ounces pita bread *or* 20 Melba
Rounds
1 tablespoon light mayonnaise
1 serving fresh fruit

OR

1 cup 1% cottage cheese *or* 8 ounces nonfat yogurt
(100–150 calories)
10 Wasa-type crackers *or* 2 ounces pita bread
or 20 Melba Rounds
1 serving fresh fruit

OR

1 frozen dinner—fewer than 320 calories, fewer than
1,100 milligrams of sodium, fewer than 11 grams of fat
1 serving fresh fruit

MIDAFTERNOON SNACK

1 medium piece fresh fruit

OR 5-ounce cup frozen nonfat yogurt (15 calories or
fewer per ounce)

OR 1 4-ounce cup nonfat regular yogurt (50-calorie
variety)

OR 1 Alba Milkshake made with water

OR 1 slice 40-calorie bread, 1 slice turkey breast, a
spread of mustard, lettuce and tomato

OR 1 slice 40-calorie bread and 1 teaspoon low-sugar jam

OR 3 Wasa-type crackers and 1 teaspoon low-sugar jam and 1 tablespoon 1% cottage cheese

OR 2 Weight Watchers' Chocolate Mousse Bars

DINNER

1½ cups cooked pasta *and* ¾ cup red spaghetti sauce
1½ cups cooked vegetables (no peas, lima beans, or corn)
Salad with fresh vegetables *and* 2 tablespoons nonfat dressing

OR

1 cup rice *and* ¾ cup lentils or beans
1½ cups cooked vegetables (no peas, lima beans, or corn)
Salad with fresh vegetables *and* 2 tablespoons nonfat dressing

OR

1 Large baked potato
2 tablespoons light sour cream
1½ cups cooked vegetables (no peas, lima beans, or corn)
Salad with fresh vegetables *and* 2 tablespoons nonfat dressing

OR

6 ounces lean fish: flounder, sole, grouper, scrod, etc.
1 medium baked potato *or* 1 cup rice *or* 1 cup cooked pasta

1½ cups cooked vegetables (no peas, lima beans, or corn)
Salad with fresh vegetables *and* 2 tablespoons nonfat dressing

OR

3 ounces skinless chicken *or* turkey *or* veal cutlet *or* salmon *or* swordfish *or* lean beef *or* lean pork (beef or pork no more often than twice a week total)
1 medium baked potato *or* 1 cup rice *or* 1 cup cooked pasta
1½ cups cooked vegetables (no peas, lima beans, or corn)
Salad with fresh vegetables *and* 2 tablespoons nonfat dressing

OR

1 frozen dinner—fewer than 320 calories, fewer than 1,100 milligrams of sodium, fewer than 11 grams of fat
1 medium roll
1½ cups cooked vegetables (no peas, lima beans, or corn)
Salad with fresh vegetables *and* 2 tablespoons nonfat dressing

EVENING SNACK
Choose 2, eat at least 1 hour apart
1 medium piece of fresh fruit
OR 1 5-ounce cup frozen nonfat yogurt (15 calories or fewer per ounce)
OR 1 4-ounce cup nonfat regular yogurt (50-calorie variety)

OR 1 Alba Milkshake made with water

OR 1 slice 40-calorie Bread, 1 slice turkey breast, a spread of mustard, lettuce and tomato

OR 1 slice 40-Calorie bread and 1 teaspoon low-sugar jam

OR 3 Wasa-type crackers and 1 teaspoon low-sugar jam and 1 tablespoon 1% cottage cheese

OR 2 Weight Watchers' Chocolate Mousse Bars

OR 2 sugar-free Fudgsicles

OR 3 cups air-popped popcorn

OR 1 cup sugar-free hot cocoa

OR ½ medium baked potato

OR 5 Melba Toasts

OR 2 cups green beans

1,200 Calories

BREAKFAST

8 ounces skim or 1% milk
¾ cup cereal, cold or cooked
1 serving fresh fruit

OR

1 egg and the white of 1 additional egg *or* 3 egg whites done in nonstick spray
1-ounce bagel (small) *or* 2 slices 40-calorie toast *or* ½ English muffin
1 serving fresh fruit

OR

⅓ cup 1% cottage cheese *or* 1 ounce 95% fat-free ham
1-ounce bagel (small) *or* 2 slices 40-Calorie toast
or ½ English muffin
1 serving fresh fruit

OR

8 ounces nonfat yogurt (100 calories)
1-ounce bagel (small) *or* 2 slices 40-calorie toast
or ½ English muffin
1 serving fresh fruit

OR

French Toast:
2 slices 40-calorie toast soaked in egg whites and skim
milk and fried in butter-flavored nonstick spray
2 tablespoons low-calorie syrup
8 ounces skim *or* 1% milk

MIDMORNING SNACK

1 medium piece fresh fruit
OR 1 4-ounce cup nonfat regular yogurt (50-calorie
     variety)
OR 1 Alba Milkshake made with water
OR 1 slice 40-calorie bread and 1 teaspoon low-sugar
     jam
OR 3 Wasa-type crackers and 1 teaspoon low-sugar
     jam and 1 tablespoon 1% cottage cheese

LUNCH
3 ounces 95–99% fat-free luncheon meat
2 slices regular bread *or* 4 slices 40-calorie bread
Lettuce and tomato
1 tablespoon light mayonnaise

OR
3 ounces water-packed tuna, salmon, *or* sardines
Large salad with raw vegetables
2 slices regular bread *or* 4 slices 40-Calorie bread
or 10 Wasa-type crackers *or* 2-ounce pita bread
or 20 Melba Rounds
1 tablespoon light mayonnaise

OR
1 cup 1% cottage cheese *or* 8 ounces nonfat yogurt
(100–150 calories)
10 Wasa-type crackers *or* 2 ounces pita bread
or 20 Melba Rounds

OR
1 frozen dinner—fewer than 320 calories, fewer than
1,100 milligrams of sodium, fewer than 11 grams of fat

MIDAFTERNOON SNACK
1 medium piece fresh fruit
OR   1 5-ounce cup frozen nonfat yogurt (15 calories or
fewer per ounce)

OR 1 4-ounce cup nonfat regular yogurt (50-calorie variety)

OR 1 Alba Milkshake made with water

OR 1 slice 40-calorie bread, 1 slice turkey breast, a spread of mustard, lettuce and tomato

OR 1 slice 40-calorie bread and 1 teaspoon low-sugar jam

OR 3 Wasa-type crackers and 1 teaspoon low-sugar jam and 1 tablespoon 1% cottage cheese

OR 2 Weight Watchers' Chocolate Mousse Bars

DINNER

1⅓ cups cooked pasta *and* ½ cup red spaghetti sauce
1½ cups cooked vegetables (no peas, lima beans, or corn)
Salad with fresh vegetables *and* 2 tablespoons nonfat dressing

OR

¾ cup rice *and* ½ cup lentils or beans
1½ cups cooked vegetables (no peas, lima beans or corn)
Salad with fresh vegetables *and* 2 tablespoons nonfat dressing

OR

1 medium baked potato
1 tablespoon light sour cream
1½ cups cooked vegetables (no peas, lima beans, or corn)
Salad with fresh vegetables *and* 2 tablespoons nonfat dressing

OR

6 ounces lean fish, flounder, sole, grouper, scrod, etc.
1 small baked potato *or* ¾ cup rice *or* ¾ cup cooked pasta
1½ cups cooked vegetables (no peas, lima beans, or corn)
Salad with fresh vegetables *and* 2 tablespoons nonfat dressing

OR

3 ounces skinless chicken *or* turkey *or* veal cutlet *or* salmon *or* swordfish *or* lean beef *or* lean pork (beef or pork no more often than twice a week total)
1 small baked potato *or* ¾ cup rice *or* ¾ cup cooked pasta
1½ cups cooked vegetables (no peas, lima beans, or corn)
Salad with fresh vegetables *and* 2 tablespoons nonfat dressing

OR

1 frozen dinner—fewer than 320 calories, fewer than 1,100 milligrams of sodium, fewer than 11 grams of fat
1½ cups cooked vegetables (no peas, lima beans, or corn)
Salad with fresh vegetables *and* 2 tablespoons nonfat dressing

EVENING SNACK
Choose 2, eat at least 1 hour apart
1 medium piece fresh fruit
OR 1 5-ounce cup frozen nonfat yogurt (15-calories or fewer per ounce)
OR 1 4-ounce cup nonfat regular yogurt (50-calorie variety)

OR 1 Alba Milkshake made with water

OR 1 slice 40-Calorie bread, 1 slice turkey breast, a
spread of mustard, lettuce and tomato

OR 1 slice 40-calorie bread and 1 teaspoon low-sugar
jam

OR 3 Wasa-type crackers and 1 teaspoon low-sugar
jam and 1 tablespoon 1% cottage cheese

OR 2 Weight Watchers' Chocolate Mousse Bars

OR 2 sugar-free Fudgsicles

OR 3 cups air-popped popcorn

OR 1 cup sugar-free hot cocoa

OR ½ medium baked potato

OR 5 Melba Toasts

OR 2 cups green beans

1000 Calories

BREAKFAST

8 ounces skim or 1% milk
¾ cup cereal, cold or cooked

OR

1 egg and the white of 1 additional egg
or 3 egg whites done in nonstick spray
1-ounce bagel (small) *or* 2 slices 40-calorie toast
or ½ English muffin

OR

⅓ cup 1% cottage cheese *or* 1 ounce 95% fat-free ham
1-ounce bagel (small) *or* 2 slices 40-calorie toast
or ½ English muffin

OR

8 ounces nonfat yogurt (100 calories)
1-ounce bagel (small) *or* 2 slices 40-calorie toast
or ½ English muffin

OR

French Toast: 1½ slices 40-calorie toast soaked in egg whites and skim milk and fried in butter-flavored nonstick spray
1 tablespoon low-calorie syrup
8 ounces skim *or* 1% milk

MIDMORNING SNACK

1 medium piece fresh fruit
OR 1 4-ounce cup nonfat regular yogurt (50-calorie variety)
OR 1 Alba Milkshake made with water
OR 1 slice 40-calorie bread and 1 teaspoon low-sugar jam
OR 3 Wasa-type crackers and 1 teaspoon low-sugar jam and 1 tablespoon 1% cottage cheese

LUNCH
3 ounces 95–99% fat-free luncheon meat
2 slices regular bread *or* 4 slices 40-calorie bread
Lettuce and tomato
1 tablespoon light mayonnaise

OR
3 ounces water-packed tuna, salmon *or* sardines
Large salad with raw vegetables
2 slices regular bread *or* 4 slices 40-calorie bread
or 10 Wasa crackers *or* 2 ounces pita bread *or* 20 Melba
Rounds
1 tablespoon light mayonnaise

OR
1 cup 1% cottage cheese *or* 8 ounces nonfat yogurt
(100–150 calories)
10 Wasa crackers *or* 2 ounces pita bread *or* 20 Melba
Rounds

OR
1 frozen dinner—fewer than 320 calories, fewer than
1,100 milligrams of sodium, fewer than 11 grams of fat

MIDAFTERNOON SNACK
1 medium piece fresh fruit
OR 1 5-ounce cup frozen nonfat yogurt (15 calories or
fewer per ounce)

OR 1 4-ounce cup non-fat regular yogurt (50-calorie variety)

OR 1 Alba Milkshake made with water

OR 1 slice 40-calorie bread, 1 slice turkey breast, a spread of mustard, lettuce and tomato

OR 1 slice 40-calorie bread and 1 teaspoon low-sugar jam

OR 3 Wasa-type crackers and 1 teaspoon low-sugar jam and 1 tablespoon 1% cottage cheese

OR 2 Weight Watchers' Chocolate Mousse Bars

DINNER

1⅓ cups cooked pasta *and* ½ cup red spaghetti sauce
1½ cups cooked vegetables (no peas, lima beans, or corn)
Salad with fresh vegetables *and* 2 tablespoons nonfat dressing

OR

¾ cup rice *and* ½ cup lentils or beans
1½ cups cooked vegetables (no peas, lima beans, or corn)
Salad with fresh vegetables *and* 2 tablespoons nonfat dressing

OR

1 medium baked potato
1 tablespoon light sour cream
1½ cups cooked vegetables (no peas, lima beans, or corn)
Salad with fresh vegetables *and* 2 tablespoons nonfat dressing

OR

6 ounces lean fish, flounder, sole, grouper, scrod, etc.
1 small baked potato *or* ¾ cup rice *or* ¾ cup cooked pasta
1½ cups cooked vegetables (no peas, lima beans, or corn)
Salad with fresh vegetables *and* 2 tablespoons nonfat dressing

OR

3 ounces skinless chicken *or* turkey *or* veal cutlet *or* salmon *or* swordfish *or* lean beef *or* lean pork (beef or pork no more often than twice a week total)
1 small baked potato *or* ¾ cup rice *or* ¾ cup cooked pasta
1½ cups cooked vegetables (no peas, lima beans, or corn)
Salad with fresh vegetables *and* 2 tablespoons nonfat dressing

OR

1 frozen dinner—fewer than 320 calories, fewer than 1,100 milligrams of sodium, fewer than 11 grams of fat
1½ cups cooked vegetables (no peas, lima beans, or corn)
Salad with fresh vegetables *and* 2 tablespoons nonfat dressing

EVENING SNACK
Choose 1 and add 1 cup diet gelatin
1 medium piece fresh fruit
OR 1 5-ounce cup frozen nonfat Yogurt (15 calories or fewer per ounce)
OR 1 4-ounce cup nonfat regular yogurt (50-calorie variety)

OR 1 Alba Milkshake made with water

OR 1 slice 40-Calorie bread, 1 slice turkey breast, a spread of mustard, lettuce and tomato

OR 1 slice 40-calorie bread and 1 teaspoon low-sugar jam

OR 3 Wasa-type crackers and 1 teaspoon low-sugar jam and 1 tablespoon 1% Cottage Cheese

OR 2 Weight Watchers' Chocolate Mousse Bars

OR 2 sugar-free Fudgsicles

OR 3 cups air-popped popcorn

OR 1 cup sugar-free hot cocoa

OR ½ medium baked potato

OR 5 melba toasts

OR 2 cups green beans

Day 13 Assignment: Write a realistic snack plan for tomorrow. This should not be too difficult if you have been keeping your daily food records. Remember, no snack attacks. Plan those snacks!

WORKSHEET

Meal Plan

BREAKFAST

MIDMORNING SNACK

LUNCH

MIDAFTERNOON SNACK

DINNER

EVENING SNACK

14

A Word About High Cholesterol and Other Ailments

At the beginning of this book, you wrote down many reasons why you want to gain control of your eating habits and lose weight. Specific health problems may have been among the reasons, and if so, they were likely ranked as highly important. What follows are brief descriptions of cholesterol, diabetes, heartburn, hiatal hernias, and a few of the myths and misunderstandings that surround them concerning diet.

Cholesterol. It is still a widely discussed and misunderstood subject. In the recent past we have heard that oat bran is good for reducing cholesterol and then that it has no positive effect. We have heard that margarine lowers cholesterol and then that it raises cholesterol. Individuals feel that whatever they are told today will be reversed tomorrow.

In the past four years I have counseled many individuals with high cholesterol. I have seen reductions in cholesterol levels of over 100 points in just one month due to dietary changes alone. In these four years, I have not changed my views in dealing with cholesterol from a dietary standpoint. And based on these views and recommendations, 80 percent of my clients have lowered their cholesterol by 20 percent or more.

When a client enters my office for nutritional counseling because he has high cholesterol, I assume that he thinks he already knows the solutions to his problem. I make that assumption because it is impossible to pick up a magazine or newspaper these days without seeing an article about cholesterol and diet. Therefore, I tell him that I'm going to make two statements that will shock him into listening to me. First: "If a product says that it has 'no cholesterol' in it, 80 percent of the time it's bad for you." Second: "I am not fond of chicken. I do not consider it a diet food."

The latter statement will be discussed in the next chapter. The first statement requires you to understand what is meant by "no cholesterol." Animal products are the only source of cholesterol in your diet. Only animals inherently have cholesterol, which is a waxy fatty substance present in their bodies. When it gets into your diet, your body may deposit it in your arteries, which will cause clogging. Plants do not contain cholesterol but they often contain fat—either saturated or unsaturated. Fat in your diet, especially saturated fat, can cause your body to *produce* cholesterol and deposit it in your arteries. Therefore, when a product claims to have no cholesterol, it means only that it contains no animal fat. It usually has a great deal of vegetable fat, perhaps even the ultrasaturated coconut oil or palm oil, although this is rare now. The *only* foods you should avoid on the basis of their cholesterol content are egg yolks, liver and other organ meats, and, to some degree, shrimp and lobster. Everything else you limit or avoid should be on the basis of its fat content. It is true that saturated fats (those that are more solid at room temperature) will elevate cholesterol more than will polyunsaturated or monounsaturated fat (those that are more liquid at room temperature and have a different chemical composition). That is why it is better to use margarine that lists *liquid* fat as the first ingredient, and why olive oil may be the oil of choice, in terms of cholesterol. **But you miss the point if you focus on the type of fat used while not making every attempt to reduce all the fat in your diet.**

I have always argued that reducing fat in the diet, losing weight, and exercising will result in lower cholesterol levels. It should be noted that in dietary terms, fat is fat. This means that the grams of fat and the calories are the same regardless of whether they come from butter, margarine, or oil.

There was at one time much discussion over whether fish oils would lower cholesterol. Omega-3 fatty acids were said to lower LDL cholesterol (the bad stuff). These oils were taken in the form of foul-smelling capsules, so people were more than glad to stop taking them when their efficacy was questioned. Whether they work is still a mystery, though more evidence appears to say no. I've never recommended the capsules because they add too much fat to the diet.

Then came the suggestion that olive oil was good for cholesterol. I never bought this one and still don't. Recommending any fat in the diet is, again, a mistake. Studies of Greeks and Italians, who eat high-fat diets but have a much lower incidence of heart disease, led researchers to study olive oil and conclude its effectiveness in lowering cholesterol. The chemical composition of the fat in olive oil—monounsaturated fatty acids—is thought to be the key. There are still two things that bother me about this. First, Greeks and Italians don't eat as much animal products as Americans do; therefore, the olive oil is the main source of fat in their diet. As already stated, animal products are the number-one source of fat in the American diet. The second problem with recommending olive oil is the way in which we use it. In Italy, olive oil sits on the table and bread is dunked into it. In America, however, we cook with it. By heating the oil we change its composition, therefore rendering it ineffective.

Now for the margarine controversy. People were originally told that as long as they ate margarine instead of butter, they were lowering their cholesterol because margarine had no cholesterol and far less saturated fat than butter. Then there was a report that proclaimed the saturated fat in margarine was more harmful than butter. My belief has always been that you may as well eat butter instead of margarine. That way, you know you are doing something wrong and will be more careful to keep the portion tiny. In this way I give clients options regarding their use of added fats. Note that if you do use margarine, the word *liquid* should precede the word *fat* on the label. It probably is helpful to use a low-calorie margarine, even though these products are lower in calories because air and water are whipped into them. Thus, you will consume fewer calories per teaspoon, unless you compensate by using more than you normally would.

My final problem in looking at any fat and its effect on cholesterol is the commonly used tunnel-vision approach. By looking at fat and its relationship to cholesterol without taking into account how fat adversely affects a variety of other ailments (including obesity, hypertension, diabetes, stomach disorders, and so on), we are not seeing a complete picture.

Remember that the fat content in your diet is the most important aspect in lowering your cholesterol and weight. Getting your fat consumption under control along with exercise will result in the best diet to help you achieve a desired cholesterol level. HDL cholesterol (the good stuff) should number 40 or greater, and is elevated only with exercise, weight loss, and quitting smoking. Diet, if anything, will lower HDL rather than raise it.

Another controversial health problem that concerns your diet is **diabetes**. This disease of the pancreas (the organ that produces insulin) has long been controlled by the use of reduced-carbohydrate diets. Fat and protein were not as restricted. Recently I had a client who had been diabetic for many years. When I began to educate him on the diet

I wanted him to follow, I first mentioned his fat consumption. (He was prone to eating large quantities of steak and butter.) He immediately got defensive and told me he had received several diet instructions that had not focused on fat at all. He then asked me where I had gotten my degree!

Fat does have a negative effect on diabetes. It appears that fat interferes with receptors in the body responsible for getting the excess sugar out of the bloodstream. The reduction of fat in the diet, even with slight liberalization of the carbohydrate, can improve blood-sugar levels. Because fat has more than twice the calories of carbohydrates, foods high in fat are packed with calories. Reducing fat, therefore, provides more quantity of carbohydrate foods.

One of the biggest cautions in advising a diet for diabetics is to guard against sugar-free items. This relates particularly to unplanned snacking. Items claiming to be void of sugar are lacking only sucrose (table sugar). They may have loads of concentrated fruit juice used as a sweetener, which can elevate blood-sugar levels as much as regular sugar does.

Snacking for diabetics should be carefully planned, for it can have a significant impact on control of blood sugar.

Heartburn is that burning-stomach sensation you may have felt and tried to relieve with antacids. Heartburn often occurs alone or as one of the symptoms of a **hiatal hernia,** in which part of the stomach protrudes through the diaphragm. With hiatal hernias, besides burning and pain, there is often pressure and the reflux of stomach acid back up the esophagus and into the back of the throat.

I found the right treatment for heartburn and hiatal hernias by accident. When cutting fat intake as part of their weight-loss programs, patients began to report to me that their stomach problems were significantly improved.

Fat is a key in the treatment of these two ailments. Because fat is more slowly digested, it stays in the stomach longer. Therefore, the irritating stomach acid has more time in which to create more pain and discomfort and to enhance the likelihood of reflux. It is important to reduce fat at dinner and afterward, as these ailments are particularly frequent at night.

Eating smaller, more frequent meals is also helpful in treating heartburn and hiatal hernias. By better metabolizing your food, you also ensure that you do not leave your stomach completely empty and thereby create additional acid.

Many health problems can be prevented or at least improved through proper nutrition. Because a low-fat diet is indicated treatment in all of them, it is unlikely that we will ever reverse the recommendation of cutting down on fat consumption for the rest of your life.

Day 14 Assignment: If you do not know your cholesterol level, make an appointment with your doctor to have it checked. Make a plan to reduce the fat in your snacks according to the recommendations in the previous chapters. Do another assessment of your recent food diaries and check for fat content. Reduce the average amount of fat you have been consuming by 25% in the next three days. Within two weeks, your snacks in total should contain less than 6 grams of fat.

WORKSHEET

My cholesterol level is: _____

My usual fat intake from snacks is: _____

Reduced by 25%, this would be: _____

To accomplish this, I will:

1. _____

2. _____

3. _____

Example:

My cholesterol level is: *235*

My usual fat intake from snacks is: *12 grams*

Reduced by 25%, this would be: *9 grams*

To accomplish this, I will:

1. Avoid candy in the afternoon

2. Switch to nonfat frozen yogurt at night in place of ice milk

3. Not put margarine on any bread products at the morning snack

15

Chicken: It's Not the Diet Food You Think It Is

Wow! That title is a shocker, isn't it? One statement I make to clients regarding diet and cholesterol is: "I am not fond of chicken. I do not consider it a diet food."

This is quite disconcerting to my clients, as most of them have eaten so much chicken for the last several years that they are about to grow feathers. For the most part, these people have completely given up red meat, thinking it was the main problem in their diet.

I have two problems with chicken. First, today we raise chicken that is much fattier than it used to be, so even when people buy skinless chicken, it still has a great deal of fat stuck to it. Second, when chicken is eaten at a restaurant and has been prepared with the skin on, even if the skin is removed before consumption, some of the fat may have dripped into the flesh. One study has disputed this theory, but in general the skin of the chicken is extremely fatty and when prepared in a restaurant it will offer temptation you could do without. When the skin of the chicken is seasoned or sauced, it becomes even more tempting. Prepared in these ways, chicken sometimes becomes as high in fat content as is lean red meat.

Because we are so busy patting ourselves on the backs for eating chicken instead of red meat, the quantity eaten is often greatly in excess of what it should be. In addition, our obsession with chicken can lead to such a lack of variety that bingeing becomes almost inevitable.

If chicken is not the answer, should we return to red meat? The answer to that is both yes and no. In other words, there was never a need to completely give up red meat. As with all animal products, it is a matter of quantity and frequency. Following are examples of how to get the optimum protein with the minimum fat.

The average person needs about 60 grams of protein each day. Only half of this needs to come from an animal source; the balance can be derived from starches and vegetables. Strict vegetarians get their protein from combining vegetable sources of protein in such a way that they do not become deficient. However, I will limit this discussion to those who consume some animal product or by-product daily.

Although the daily protein requirement is 60 grams, the average person eats about 100 grams of protein each day. My objection to high amounts of protein in the diet is that its source is primarily animal products. Economically, it is also a waste of money. Why pay four dollars per pound for skinless chicken for dinner—a meal at which you need calories, not protein—when you can buy pasta at seventy-nine cents per pound?

Last, high amounts of protein over a long period of time create an additional strain on the kidneys, which could eventually create problems in some individuals. There is really no need to overconsume protein, but because we have been programmed to do so, it takes time to change.

Remember to use the 2-2-2-1 rule for dinner (see chapter 12), and try to keep the protein selections for breakfast and lunch to very lean choices. The following material will help you further lower your protein intake without feeling deprived. As stated earlier, it is important to make changes gradually when you are attached to a particular behavior. Anything you do for the sake of a diet will be short-lived, and you are now interested only in permanent changes.

Let's start with egg whites. There, nature created the perfect low-calorie high-protein food. It's a shame it was put together with such a high-cholesterol, high-fat food—the yolk. At first, egg whites may seem unappealing, but there are several interesting ways to enjoy them. The white of an egg provides only 15 calories and 4 grams of protein. This is in contrast to the yolk, which yields 60 calories and 5 grams of fat.

Try scrambling the whites with onions, mushrooms, peppers, and chives for a colorful, tasteful omelet. Cook it in a nonstick-sprayed pan, and fill it with low-fat cottage cheese, farmer's cheese, or salsa. Use egg whites with skim milk and cinnamon as a dipping for diet French toast: simply fry it in a nonstick-sprayed pan and serve with a little low-calorie syrup. Both of these are excellent choices for breakfast or for terrific nontraditional lunches.

1% cottage cheese is another excellent source of protein that provides minimal calories and fat. The specific analysis: 1 cup equals 164 calories, only 2 grams of fat, and a whopping 28 grams of protein. Even though the fat content is low, we still want to limit protein, so 1 cup is too much at one time. Limit each serving to ½ cup.

Cottage cheese makes an excellent entrée when mixed with noodles and either eaten that way or baked with Italian seasoning and marinara sauce. Hot lunches are often a monotony breaker to the routine sandwich and such a baked meal adds variety.

For breakfast, spread cottage cheese on a slice of toast and sprinkle it with cinnamon. This tastes like a Danish pastry.

Even if you don't like baked fish, consider the possibilities for cold fish, especially shellfish, as a lean and filling lunch. This includes the new varieties of imitation crab, which are usually made from pollack, another extremely low-fat fish. This means the crab salad served in restaurants is usually a safer choice than the tuna salad, because the crab or imitation crab is leaner than tuna. Also, the crab salad is a little more watery and therefore the mayonnaise tends to drip away from the crab rather than stick together as with tuna salad.

How about a shrimp cocktail for lunch? It's very low

in fat, it sticks with you, and if you don't add too much cocktail sauce, you won't be adding too many extra calories. A 3-ounce portion of shrimp has 78 calories, less than 1 gram of fat, and 16 grams of protein.

The new nonfat yogurts make great breakfasts and lunches. There are varieties that come prepared with fruit and sweetener; or, if you prefer, eat the plain nonfat yogurt and mix in your own fruit and a sweetener.

Have you ever tried yogurt cheese? It tastes like cream cheese but has no fat. To make it, simply line a strainer or colander with cheesecloth and pour in the yogurt. Place over a bowl to catch the drippings and refrigerate overnight. The next day, discard the drippings and use the yogurt cheese as a replacement for cream cheese.

Last, since chicken is probably a big part of your life now, the following are some healthful ways of eating it. Chicken should be eaten only when prepared without any skin or fat. Cutting the chicken into small pieces will keep the portion to 3 ounces or less.

For one of my favorite chicken dishes, take leftover noodles, fresh chopped vegetables, and leftover or fresh chicken and stir-fry in a pan or wok treated with nonstick spray.

Another tasty dish can be made by topping your salad with strips of grilled chicken, hot or cold, and lots of fresh vegetables. Eat the salad this way or stuff it into a pita pocket. An ounce of chicken, like most meat, fish, or other poultry, has about 7 grams of protein and anywhere from 3 to 6 grams of fat per ounce. So the portion should always be limited to 3 ounces or less. It takes time, but trying these and other new dishes should make a bit easier the transition to a diet lower in fat and containing less animal products.

Day 15 Assignment: Identify the foods you typically rely on for protein. Are you a protein overeater? Cut down the protein in your snacks by 25 percent in the next three days. Within the next two weeks you should eliminate protein from your snacks unless they contain 1 gram of fat or less.

WORKSHEET

My current protein intake for snacks is: _____

Reduced by 25 percent, this is: _____

To reduce this quantity, I will:

1. _____

2. _____

3. _____

Example:

My current protein intake for snacks is: *7 grams*

Reduced by 25 percent, this is: *5 grams*

To reduce this quantity, I will:

1. Not eat nuts except at a party once a month
2. Not have a stacked sandwich as the evening snack
3. Switch to 1% cottage cheese so I can use it as a morning snack and it will have less than 1 gram of fat

16

Pasta Power

You can lose weight by eating more spaghetti. Surprised? Most people believe that spaghetti is fattening. And in many cases, they're correct. When it is loaded with meat and/or sausage or when the sauce has a high amount of oil, and all is consumed with a ton of buttered garlic bread, it can have many more calories than a big steak dinner. But when your palate learns to appreciate spaghetti and other pasta dishes in a new manner, your menu will have new variety and appeal. It is also very motivating to suddenly lose weight on an entrée that you once considered extremely fattening.

Furthermore, we now understand that the body burns carbohydrate better than it burns fat. Since spaghetti can be eaten with relatively little fat, as opposed to most of the other dinner entrées, the body will burn it more efficiently. This is most important at night, when our metabolism is apt to be at its lowest level. Think about it: even if you don't exercise (and you should be doing so by now), you are undoubtedly more active during the day than in the evening. Therefore, the pasta works best at dinner.

Because a pasta meal has little protein, it important to remember the basics of the recommended meal plan. When having a dinner that is low in protein, it is essential to have consumed adequate protein earlier in the day. That means protein at breakfast (such as milk, yogurt, an egg, or cottage cheese) and at lunch (turkey breast, tuna, ground turkey, lean luncheon meats, and so on). Having done that, you can safely have a low-protein dinner. If you haven't had adequate protein by dinner and you plan to have pasta, drink a glass of skim milk to get the needed protein.

One of the things people like most about pasta for dinner is its simplicity! We often dread dieting because we anticipate a great deal more preparation than we wish to do. Most diets call for more salads, fresh vegetables, and entrées that require additional work. Spaghetti, on the other hand, requires boiling, and that's it! Cooked, drained pasta can be kept in the refrigerator for about four days. The sauce, homemade or commercial, can be kept in the refrigerator for a week or more and freezes well. So, you can make large batches of pasta and sauce, and subsequent dinners will require only brief microwaving of sauce or boiling of new pasta and throwing a salad together.

How can a commercial sauce be used when the meal is a pasta marinara? There are two choices. The first is to purchase a sauce prepared without oil (read the ingredients label to make sure). The other option is to dilute a commercial sauce that contains oil by adding extra tomatoes and other vegetables. For example:

A commercial sauce states that it has 5 grams of fat per 4-ounce serving. This is too much. Take the 32-ounce jar of sauce and pour it into a large pitcher or other container. Add to this a 28-ounce can of whole tomatoes, including the juice. In a pan sprayed with nonstick coating, sauté mushrooms, onions, garlic, peppers, and zucchini in any amount desired, then add the vegetables to the sauce. If the sauce tastes a bit acidic, add artificial sweetener.

This process will more than double the original volume of sauce, so that that the "doctored" sauce now has fewer than 2.5 grams of fat per 4-ounce serving—a much more acceptable level.

Another advantage to pasta and other high-carbohydrate foods is that they seem to satisfy people's cravings for sweets. Thus, control of eating becomes much easier. You will begin to notice that you have less desire for dessert after a pasta dinner than after more traditional dinners.

As mentioned in the assignment for this chapter (p. 140), spaghetti marinara should not be the only type of pasta meal you consume. There is much variety in pasta, and often other entrées make use of pasta leftovers. This will save you time in the kitchen! The following recipe counts as a stir-fry, no-oil dinner in your 2-2-2-1 meal plan:

> Spray a pan with nonstick coating and place over medium heat. Put in leftover chicken in the amount of 3 ounces or fewer per person. Add any leftover pasta (about ¾ cup cooked per person) or cook pasta to a slightly underdone stage (rotini works well here). Add any leftover vegetables or throw in mushrooms, broccoli, carrots, snow peas, and so on. Stir-fry with a splash of wine or low-sodium soy sauce.

The pasta meal most difficult to duplicate while keeping the fat content low is pasta with garlic and olive oil. There is simply nothing that can imitate the oil and yield the same flavor and texture. Your best bet is to try adding more garlic in its own juice and to use an olive-oil-flavored nonstick spray placed directly onto the pasta. Another option is to use a no-fat butter/margarine substitute that you reconstitute with water. This will give the taste of butter without the calories.

If you wish to have a pasta dish for lunch, just remember to add some protein. When using the leftover spaghetti marinara, add 2 ounces of ground turkey. If you eat the chicken pasta dish, you already have enough protein.

Now that you have your heart set on pasta and its power to help you lose weight and gain control of your eating habits, let's discuss portions. This is an essential detail because even though pasta burns better than entrées that contain more fat, you cannot double the calories you consume. The bottom line in losing weight is that you must take in fewer calories than your body burns.

Does this mean that you have to begin that tedious task of weighing and measuring everything that goes in your mouth? Yes and no. Yes, in the sense that it's helpful to realize just how much the recommended portion is. But no, in the sense that consistently weighing food is integral only to dieting and will not help you control your food habits for life. Weighing or measuring portions a few times will let you know what the portion looks like on the plates you normally use.

A client complained that she was enjoying her pasta too much and therefore found it almost impossible to control her portions. I asked her to measure the portion of spaghetti that I recommended, then to cut it in half and refrigerate it. She was to serve the first portion of spaghetti with her salad and vegetable as usual, and an hour later, whether she was hungry or not, heat up the other half of the spaghetti and eat it. I guaranteed her that for at least that night, she would be able to control her portion. I also told her that if she repeated this new behavior each time she ate spaghetti, she would eventually lose her desire to eat the second portion. This proves that portion control is greatly a mental exercise.

Additional help in controlling your portions of pasta comes from eating large amounts of cooked vegetables with the meal. Think of it this way: a 10-ounce box of frozen green beans contains about 75 calories—less than ½ cup of cooked pasta. When I think in these terms, I can see myself consuming the pasta in one gulp. That would be impossible with the green beans, which take considerably longer and would be more filling.

So, to enjoy the true benefit of pasta power, make sure you eat your vegies. You'll be on your way to controlling your portions as a part of your new eating behavior, which includes avoiding snack attacks.

Day 16 Assignment: Try pasta in a new way. If you have been eating spaghetti marinara for the vegetarian dinners, try a new recipe. It is important that you don't get tired of having the same meals. Notice that during the nights when you have had a vegetarian dinner, you are no more likely to have a snack attack than during the nights when you eat a more traditional dinner. That is because eating after dinner has little to do with hunger and much to do with habit, boredom, and the like.

WORKSHEET

My new pasta dish is: _____

In looking back over my food diaries, I have stayed in control of my night snacking _____ of _____ days when I have had a vegetarian dinner

Example:

My new pasta dish is: pasta, sautéed in butter-flavored nonstick spray with minced garlic

In looking back over my food diaries, I have stayed in control of my night snacking *10* of *12* days when I have had a vegetarian dinner

———————————————————————————

17

Fiber and Rain

*A*re you confused by the title of this chapter? The importance of a high-fiber diet will be stressed here, as well as the necessity of a good water intake. The two must go hand in hand, and the reasons for this will be clarified throughout the chapter.

What is your current fiber intake? Chances are, you don't know. The typical American diet contains about 8 grams of fiber, although 25 grams is a more appropriate number. Fiber comes from a variety of sources, including whole-grain cereals and breads, vegetables, fruits, beans, lentils, and legumes.

Among the many attributes of fiber is that it improves bowel regularity and provides relief from constipation. This is accomplished by the digestible and indigestible particles of fiber pulling water into the colon, making the stool softer and easier to pass.

Because of this, incidence of colon cancer is reduced.

Some experts feel that when the fecal material moves through the colon more rapidly, the organisms that would likely cause cancer have less of a chance to irritate the colon. Over the past fifty years, while the consumption of cereal and other fibers has decreased, the incidence of colon cancer has proportionately increased.

Diverticular disease is the protrusion of pockets into the intestinal tract. This can be a painful condition when material collects in these pockets. In extreme situations surgery may be required, which always poses a risk to health. A high-fiber diet reduces the likelihood of developing diverticular disease.

Fiber found in beans, oats, and fruits may have the ability to lower cholesterol and thereby reduce the risk of heart disease. Additionally, these same fibers may lower insulin requirements among diabetics.

Are you convinced yet? Let's review a few more benefits having more to do with helping you conquer your cravings.

First, there are parts of fiber that are not digestible. That means there are no calories associated with eating portions of these foods. This may reduce the total number of calories in a particular food. Fiber can fill the stomach because it increases bulk. It also delays the emptying of the stomach, which creates a feeling of fullness for a longer period of time. This fullness will at least take care of the physical basis of the desire for unplanned snacks.

Eaten before a meal, high-fiber foods can make it almost impossible for you to consume a large quantity of the meal. And because most fiber is contained in starchy foods and vegetables, it helps regulate your diet by leaving far less room for fat calories.

You may object to eating a high-fiber diet since it can cause an increased amount of intestinal gas and lower-abdominal discomfort. That is often the side effect of a high-fiber diet embarked upon too quickly. If your diet contains only 6 grams of fiber today, it is not appropriate to increase it to 25 grams tomorrow. This should be done slowly and with a gradual increase in water intake.

Earlier I stated that fiber draws water into the colon to promote elimination. It therefore makes sense that there must be a great deal of water in the diet to accomplish this. A high-fiber diet can actually constipate you if there is not sufficient water in your diet. Without it, all the undigested material becomes dry and hard to pass through the colon.

Water is responsible for more than half of your body weight. It therefore makes sense to replace some of that water on a daily basis. Water levels in the body are affected by a variety of factors. Women, because of their hormonal cycles, are subject to wide fluctuations in water balance. Salt intake affects the amount of water anyone's body retains.

The best way to rid the body of excess retained water is to drink *more* water. When the individual senses he is retaining fluid, then cuts back on his water intake to compensate, the body responds by retaining more fluid. Remember that by cutting back on water intake, you will cause an opposite reaction.

Water drunk before a meal, or virtually anytime, tends to send a signal to the brain that the stomach has something in it. This can temporarily reduce the craving for an unplanned snack, and sometimes that is all you will need to conquer a craving.

Water is present to some degree in almost every food and beverage we consume. Some foods such as lettuce, fruits, and vegetables are higher in water content than foods such as meats, poultry, breads, and pasta. But when we discuss increasing our water intake, we mean water, pure and simple.

When I stated that the body is composed primarily of water, I meant *water*. That does not include tea, coffee, diet soda, juice, or any other natural or unnatural beverage. Water, plain seltzer, and bottled or distilled water are the only beverages you can include as part of the 80 ounces (ten 8-ounce glasses) I recommend you drink daily.

You will also achieve a certain mental discipline by drinking water. Most people don't like to drink 80 ounces a day, so, in having to do so, you will be training your mind at the same time you replenish your body. Remember that by increasing the amount of water you drink you will feel better when you gradually increase the fiber in your diet.

FIBER CONTENT OF FOODS

PRODUCT	SERVING SIZE	GRAMS OF FIBER
CEREALS AND GRAINS		
All Bran Extra	½ cup	13
Fiber One Cereal	½ cup	12
Whole-wheat pasta	1 cup cooked	5
Bran flakes	½ cup	4
Raisin bran	½ cup	4
Whole-wheat bread	1 slice	2
Light bread (40 calories)	1 slice	2
Cheerios	1 ounce	2
Grapenuts	¼ cup	2
Oatmeal	1 ounce	2
Popcorn	1 cup	2
Pumpernickle bread	1 slice	1
Rye bread	1 slice	1
Brown rice	½ cup	†
White rice	½ cup	†
Pasta	½ cup	†

† = Less than 1 gram of fiber

PRODUCT	SERVING SIZE	GRAMS OF FIBER
COOKED LEGUMES		
Kidney beans	½ cup	9
Baked beans	½ cup	7
Navy beans	½ cup	5
Pinto beans	½ cup	5
Lentils	½ cup	2
VEGETABLES		
Frozen peas	½ cup	4
Baked potato w/skin	1 medium	4
Cooked broccoli tops	½ cup	3
Cooked young carrots	½ cup	3
Cooked corn	½ cup	3
Cooked green beans	½ cup	2
Brussels sprouts	½ cup	2
Cooked eggplant	½ cup	2
Cooked sweet potato	½ medium	2
Red cabbage	½ cup	2
Raw bean sprouts	½ cup	1
Raw lettuce	½ cup	1
Raw mushrooms	½ cup	1
Fresh tomato	½ medium	1
Dill pickel	1 medium	1

PRODUCT	SERVING SIZE	GRAMS OF FIBER
FRUITS AND NUTS		
Almonds	¼ cup	5*
Dried prunes	3	4**
Apple w/skin	1 medium	3
Banana	1 medium	3**
Blackberries	½ cup	3
Dried dates	5	3**
Nectarine	1 medium	3
Peach w/skin	1 medium	3
Peanuts	¼ cup	3*
Strawberries	1 cup	3
Cantaloupe	¼ cup	2
Orange	1 medium	2
Tangerine	1 medium	2
Walnuts	¼ cup	2*
Apricot	1 medium	1
Cherries	10 large	1**
Grapefruit	½ medium	1
Pineapple	½ cup	1
Raisins	2 tablespoons	1**

* = High-fat and -calorie food
** = High-calorie food

Day 17 Assignment: Take one of your planned snacks and add 3 grams of fiber to it. Make sure to write in your food diary and note the example below for a revised version, which includes recording your daily exercise and the amount of time you spend doing it. Make sure you record your water intake. You should start working on gradually increasing your water intake to 80 ounces daily. Drink most of this between meals.

WORKSHEET

Food Diary

FOOD	TIME OF DAY	PLACE	WITH WHOM	GRAMS OF FAT

Example: (continue to record all intake)

FOOD	TIME OF DAY	PLACE	WITH WHOM	GRAMS OF FAT
8 ounces skim milk	7:00 A.M.	Kitchen	Alone	1 Gram

Fiber and Rain

FOOD	TIME OF DAY	PLACE	WITH WHOM	GRAMS OF FAT
¾ cup cereal				0 Grams
½ cup berries				
Water: 32 ounces				
Exercise: stationary biking 30 minutes				

18

Eat Before You Eat

In still another attempt to gain better control of your eating habits, try eating before you eat. Few people escape realizing that part of the reason they overconsume is that they eat too fast. They go from feeling starved to feeling stuffed without having experienced that just-satisfied feeling in between. This rapid-eating pattern starts early in life and is reinforced throughout by our mobile, eat-on-the-run society. The problem with eating too fast is that it inevitably leads to overeating.

It has been suggested that the brain and the stomach have a communication process whereby the stomach sends a signal to the brain when it has been satisfied. The problem is that this signal does not occur until about twenty minutes after the person has begun eating. Since many of our meals don't last twenty minutes, overeating and the stuffed feeling often occur.

Thus, the appetite-suppressing action of food occurs when

you consume a small portion of bulky food that is low in calories. If you do this twenty minutes before the start of the actual meal, the signal will hit your brain just as you sit down at the table. That will make it easier for you to consume a smaller portion of food and still feel satisfied.

Another advantage to eating a snack before a meal is that it keeps you from beginning the meal when you are starving. The worst time to eat is when you are desperately hungry, because you will tend to overeat. Your brain may have received the hunger signal from your stomach for so long that it will be hard to stop eating after a normal portion.

Manufacturers in the diet industry have tried to capitalize on the idea of eating before you eat by providing products that fill you up when taken before a meal. Do you remember the fiber tablets that were so heavily advertised? You took two of them and a large glass of water before a meal, and that was supposed to fill you up. Well, I took one of those pills and dropped it into a cup of water. It sank to the bottom of the glass and dissolved into what looked like a half-teaspoon of dirt. I couldn't see why that would have any ability to suppress the appetite. And experts agreed, stating that these pills were useless. What *was* useful was the glass of water that was drunk with the tablets, for it provided the full feeling experienced. Additionally, the tablets may have provided psychological benefits that helped curb the appetite. In other words, when you think something will work for you, frequently it will.

The most important criterion for the eat-before-you-eat rule is that whatever you eat, it should be accompanied by water and lots of it! You experience an automatic feeling of bulk in the stomach with water alone. Whether or not you decide always to have a small, filling snack before your meals, you should drink water before each meal and each snack.

The foods that will work best for these purposes are high-fiber, high-carbohydrate items. The fiber provides that extra feeling of bulk and will not empty from the stomach as quickly as do more easily digestible foods. A lean protein food will also work—if you have been careful not to have too much protein during the day.

This pre-meal snack should contain between 40 and 60 calories. That may not seem like enough to do anything, but remember, all you want is to give your brain a signal. If water alone can sometimes do that, then it will take only a small amount of food to provide the desired effect. What is essential is that you plan the item, eat the item, and stick just to that. What you don't want to do is nibble your way right into the upcoming meal.

Be sure to count these snacks into your meal plan. While the goal is to help you reduce your urge to eat large portions at a meal, the snack still has calories and these need to be counted.

The following are 40-to-60–calorie snacks that will provide bulk and a satiated feeling that should send the right signal to the brain.

FOOD	CALORIES	FIBER
½ cup Fiber One cereal	60	13
1 ounce chick peas	51	2

FOOD	CALORIES	FIBER
I cup cooked green beans	31	2
½ cup cooked peas	52	1.6
3 Melba Toast w/I teaspoon low-sugar jam	58	2
I slice 40-calorie bread w/½ ounce turkey breast	55	2
½ medium baked potato	47	.3
2 medium carrots	50	1
I cup sliced beets	45	1
4 ounces Dannon Light Yogurt	50	—
½ cup skim milk	45	—
2 Triplecracker Rye Krisp	60	.2
I cup raspberries	60	3.7
I large peach	45	1
I cup strawberries	45	.8
2 ounces shrimp	56	—
⅓ cup corn-bran cereal	49	.5
⅔ cup Cheerios	59	.2
60-calorie hot cocoa mix	60	—

That should give you sufficient options for now. Remember that it is sometimes better to plan snacks well ahead of time so that the spontaneous desire to eat does not get to you.

Also remember that we mentioned that fiber pills are not effective in suppressing appetite. However, there is a product designed for increasing the bulk in the diet that can be very effective in curbing the appetite: Metamucil. Most often taken to alleviate constipation, Metamucil when taken before a meal with the prescribed amount of water is highly effective in controlling appetite.

If you are in control of your portions at meals, you may want to use the idea of eating before you eat only for "dangerous events" such as parties, restaurants, and so on. Otherwise, if meal portions are still larger than desirable, consider trying the suggestions every day for a week before lunch and dinner. Either way, you have new ammunition to combat literally biting off more than you can chew!

Day 18 Assignment: By now you should have a better handle on when you are really hungry and when you are having a snack attack. However, one habit you may still have is consuming too much food at a meal, particularly at dinner. To accomplish better control, begin eating a 60-calorie snack twenty minutes before dinner at least twice a week. Plan for this, and write it on the sheet provided.

WORKSHEET

Meal plan for two 60-calorie snacks twice a week:

_____

_____

_____

_____

When I do this, I will eliminate:

_____

_____

_____

_____

Example:

Meal plan for two 60-calorie snacks twice a week:
Tuesday (the night I work late and walk in the door famished) I will have 1 ounce of chick peas (to reduce the temptation for nuts) and a club soda before dinner.
Friday (the night we go out) I'll have a 60-calorie milkshake, which will bloat me before a tempting dinner.

When I do this, I will eliminate:
On Tuesday, since I'm eating late anyway, I'll eliminate one of my evening snacks.
On Friday, I'll eat half the starch (bread or crackers) at lunch.

19

The Good News
About Sugar

This title may really surprise you. Most people believe that the single biggest contributor to their weight problem is sugar or sweets. People equate sugar with sweets, when actually they are not the same. The next time you think you're having a sugar craving, think of trying to satisfy it with a piece of hard candy. In all likelihood, you will say, "No, that's not what I want." What you are craving is fat—you know, something like a premium ice cream or a brownie or piece of rich chocolate candy.

There does seem to be an innate craving for sweets, and whether they are rich sweets or not, the drive to eat them creates problems. In fact, some believe that a person can crave sugar in an addictive fashion similar to that of people who abuse drugs or alcohol. This theory is based on the fact that sugar releases a chemical in the brain that makes the person feel calm and relaxed. Problems arise when the calm feeling does not last very long and the person then craves more sugar and with greater frequency to produce this feeling.

Whether this theory is true physiologically is not important. What is important is knowing whether this scenario describes how you relate to sweets. If so, you must take action to deal with the problem.

There are two distinct ways to deal with a craving for sweets. The first is the most effective and the most difficult. Of the people who will try this method, less than 1 percent will stick with it on a long-term basis. It is the cold-turkey approach to sweets. The individual decides to abstain from all sweets, sugar, and even sugar substitutes. In doing this nearly impossible task, you will notice that the craving for sweets lessens each day and virtually disappears within two weeks. The problem with this approach is that if you cheat, possibly with even one sweet indulgence, you will return to craving the sweets. Think of people you know who quit smoking, even for long periods of time. Just one cigarette gets them smoking again.

The easier and more sensible alternative is to eat sweets moderately, to your advantage. With the advent of numerous low-sugar and artificially sweetened items, this is not difficult, as long as you pay attention to calories and *fat*.

As we have discussed, fat is the most detrimental form of caloric intake, as it has more than twice the calories of carbohydrates and protein. Sugar has the same amount of calories as carbohydrates (it is itself a carbohydrate). If you doubt this, just look at a box of corn flakes and sugar-frosted flakes and you'll see that ounce for ounce the calories are the same. This does not mean it is okay to eat sugar when you have a craving for sweets. But if you are going to get in trouble, at least do it with sugar alone instead of sugar and fat.

Remember, there is evidence that we metabolize sugar and other carbohydrates more effectively than we do fat. In other words, there is thought to be a thermodynamic burn from the digestion of carbohydrate. Fat, however is believed to slow down metabolism. So when you eat carbohydrates, think of it as stoking a fire.

A few examples of where sugar works in place of fat:

- **Using jam instead of butter or margarine on toast**
- **Using a sweet marinade such as juice in place of oil for meats and chicken**

Then there are the numerous desserts that are fat-free but do have sugar or juice used as a sweetener, including cookies, frozen yogurt and other frozen desserts, muffins, and so on.

Of course, sugar substitutes lower the calories even more. But as with every other lesson in this book, a caution of moderation is still made. You may ask, what is the harm, if the calories are low enough? Consider the following example:

A man came into my office seeking a liquid-protein diet. He weighed more than 350 pounds and walked with a cane because of his weight, despite the fact that he was only fifty-three years old. He told me that he had used a liquid diet once before and had lost over 100 pounds but had eventually regained it. He said he wasn't sure how that had happened, but that when he started to eat again he would make a relish tray of carrots, celery, and the like, and whenever he wanted to eat he would eat raw vegetables.

I told him that was the beginning of the end. He was a bit mystified. How could a celery stick be harmful? he wondered. When he told himself that he could go to the kitchen and eat something anytime he wanted to, as long as it was the right food, that was a lie! The habit of nibbling is wrong, no matter what the food is, because the right food will soon turn into danger foods, due to the habit and lack of awareness. He admitted that I was right, that soon after the celery sticks lost their appeal, cheese, salami, and whole sandwiches followed.

You cannot eat *anything* you want as often as you want, regardless of the calorie content. Most overweight people want to nibble often, and this creates an unconsciousness about the eating process, which leads to a multitude of problems. Among them is the lack of satisfaction after eating, caused mostly by the guilt associated with over-consumption. This feeling is usually verbalized as, "I don't know why I even ate that, it really wasn't that good."

So, all calories count as much for habit control as calorie control. And whether it's sweets or other food, plan it, enjoy it, and control it.

Day 19 Assignment: Identify items in your food diaries that you have been nibbling on because they have few or no calories. *Stop it!* You cannot have any food in unlimited quantities. Snacking in this way is a dangerous habit. If you have fallen victim to it, make a list of activities you can do instead of eating when you feel the urge to snack at an unplanned time.

WORKSHEET

Activities Incompatible with Eating that I Can Do:

1. _____
2. _____
3. _____
4. _____
5. _____
6. _____

Example:

1. Talk on the phone (many people eat during this, but I never do)
2. Walk the dog
3. Take a long hot bath
4. Catch up on sewing
5. Write a letter
6. Pay bills—ugh!

20

Metabolism: How to Make It Work

In this chapter we will review the difference between hormonal control of metabolism (thyroid) versus the internal metabolism that no one can seem to get a handle on. A low-functioning thyroid is easily identified. Your doctor can do a blood test to determine if your thyroid gland is causing your metabolism to work too slowly. If this is the case, you will receive medication that will improve the hormonal control over your metabolism. As was stated earlier, that is the easy part.

Can you have normal thyroid function and still have a sluggish metabolism? The answer is a definite *yes*. The problem is that even if it could be positively identified (it can, but there are very few places that do this testing), the recommendation would be the same: *You must eat less and expend more energy (calories).*

People develop slow metabolisms for a variety of reasons. Certainly some people were born with this awful situation, which may in part explain their obesity. Studies have shown that there is an 80 percent chance that a child will become obese if both his parents are obese. It was always thought that the reason for this was environment. In other words, if the child saw his parents devouring lots of junk, he would learn to do the same. Therefore, he would become fat.

But in looking for another explanation for obesity, genetics became a proven factor. This was shown through studies of children who were adopted. When children were born to thin parents and then adopted by obese parents, follow-up visits years later showed that the children grew to be thin adults. Likewise, when children were born to obese parents and then adopted by thin parents, they too followed the pattern of their biologic parents and became obese. So, while environment may be a negative contributor, genetics are a strong factor. Does this mean that you are doomed to be overweight? No. But it does mean that you will have to take *every* suggestion in this chapter. You'll have to try the best you can to make your metabolism work effectively.

Yo-yo dieting—the repeated losing and regaining of weight—is certainly a cause of slow metabolism. This is evidenced by a variety of studies, including experiments that show that if a person loses weight at one caloric level the first time, he will have to cut his caloric intake substantially more the next time he attempts to lose weight. These studies also show that weight is regained at double the rate at which it is lost.

Going on a diet slows down your metabolism. As was

earlier described, the body has a strong survival instinct and interprets caloric reduction as a threat to that survival. This is true particularly when the calories are very low (usually 800 calories or fewer per day). Studies have shown examples similar to the following:

> A person consuming 600 calories per day burns 400 calories during a 45-minute stationary-bike workout as measured. The following day, the measurements show that the person burns 400 calories fewer than he did the previous day. This means his body is conserving all the energy it can because the net intake of calories is so low that there is a serious threat to survival.

While all this is pretty frustrating, there are some methods proven to speed up metabolism. While none of these alone can stimulate the body to burn calories at a greatly increased rate, in combination they can assure that the body metabolizes at its most efficient rate.

Aerobic exercise. It's worth mentioning again. Aerobic exercise will stimulate your resting metabolism. There is even evidence that there is an increase in calories burned for up to twelve hours after aerobic exercise is performed. In addition, in terms of maintenance of weight loss, exercise is absolutely essential if you want to keep your metabolism working at its optimal level.

Weight training. Different from aerobic exercise, weight training, either with free weights, isometric exercises, or weight machines such as Nautilus, will build muscle mass. There is a proportionate increase in the body's metabolic rate to the increase in muscle mass. Though not for everyone, weight training can firm up areas where fat has been lost, so now there's an even better reason to do it. This does not mean you need to look bulky. Even slight increases in muscle mass will cause some improvement in metabolism.

Eating small, frequent meals. The more often you eat, the better. If that surprises you, watch a thin person eat. Make sure it is a person who claims she doesn't have to watch her weight. This thin person seems to eat all the time. The major difference is that she rarely overeats. She will open a box of crackers and take out two, then put away the box. An hour later, she eats another small snack. Most overeaters would not even open a box of crackers if they didn't intend to eat quite a few at one sitting.

To further convince yourself that eating more often raises metabolism, review the example given in chapter 1:

> There are two groups of people in a study. One group eats one meal a day that contains 500 calories. The other group eats three meals a day totaling 1,000 calories. Using the normally accepted theory that when you have eliminated 3,500 calories from your diet, you will lose 1 pound, you would expect that the group consuming half the calories (the 500-calorie group) would lose twice as much weight, twice as fast, as the 1,000-calorie group. In reality, the two

groups lose the same amount of weight at the same rate.

Don't skip breakfast. If you are a chronic dieter, your body has learned to compensate for decreases in caloric intake by decreasing your metabolism. As earlier stated, when you don't eat breakfast, your body perceives that you are beginning a fast. It doesn't know how long you intend to go without eating, it just knows that it better slow down its calorie burning.

Breakfast with protein—i.e., skim milk, cottage cheese, or yogurt—will tell your body that you are not going to starve yourself. The protein is essential because it is digested more slowly and released more gradually into the bloodstream. This gives a better metabolic burning process than carbohydrate alone, which empties from the stomach rapidly and may send the wrong messages to the brain regarding metabolism.

Consume a low-fat diet. This point can't be reiterated too often: Carbohydrate burns more efficiently than fat. There is a better burning that fuels the metabolism when a low-fat diet is followed. The fact that eating fat makes us fat seems to make sense to most people, but the evidence to support this concept is fairly new.

Furthermore, a low-fat diet contains more food because the caloric density of the foods is so much less. So, if you want to eat more and make your metabolism work better, eat a low-fat diet.

The desire and motivation to lose weight and to maintain

that loss are your keys to success. Getting your metabolism in optimal working order and keeping it that way are important steps in preventing the frustration commonly experienced by chronic dieters. These tools will allow you to begin eating in a controlled fashion and to stop labeling yourself a ''dieter.''

Day 20 Assignment: Analyze your recent food records. Make sure that at least 500 calories are eaten daily by 3:00 P.M. This amount may be divided between meals and snacks.

WORKSHEET

Food Diary

BREAKFAST **BREAKFAST CALORIES:**

_____

_____

_____

MIDMORNING
SNACK **SNACK CALORIES:**

_____

LUNCH **LUNCH CALORIES:**

_____

_____

_____

_____

MIDAFTERNOON   SNACK CALORIES:
SNACK

_____

DINNER   DINNER CALORIES:

_____

_____

_____

EVENING SNACK   SNACK CALORIES:

_____

_____

Calories Eaten Before 3:00 P.M.
Calories Eaten After 3:00 P.M.

Example:

BREAKFAST   BREAKFAST CALORIES: 230

1 egg and the white of 1 additional egg
done in nonstick spray
2 slices 40-calorie toast
1 apple

MIDMORNING SNACK   SNACK CALORIES: 50

4-ounce cup of nonfat regular yogurt (50-calorie variety)

LUNCH   LUNCH CALORIES: 335

3 ounces water-packed tuna
Large salad with raw vegetables
2 slices regular bread
1 tablespoon light mayonnaise

MIDAFTERNOON SNACK   SNACK CALORIES: 60

1 medium piece fresh fruit

DINNER   DINNER CALORIES: 445

1⅓ cups cooked pasta *and* ½ cup red spaghetti sauce
1½ cups cooked vegetables (no peas, lima beans, or corn)
Salad with fresh vegetables *and* 2 tablespoons
nonfat dressing

EVENING SNACK   SNACK CALORIES: 120

1 slice 40-calorie bread and 1 teaspoon low-sugar jam
2 Weight Watchers' Chocolate Mousse Bars

Calories before 3:00 P.M.: 675
Calories after 3:00 P.M.: 565

21

Just Do It

The preceding chapter provided an explanation of how metabolism works and how to make it work better. The methods suggested there are excellent for improving your metabolism to whatever degree you can. The following suggestions will improve your daily caloric expenditure and increase your feeling of control over your life. This chapter describes what "lifestyle activity" is and how you can make it work for you.

Most people, overweight or not, take the easy way out. We have become a society of couch potatoes and are lazier than ever. These facts are evident despite the growing awareness of health issues. Less than 40 percent of American adults engage in aerobic exercise (that is, twenty minutes or longer, at least three times a week). The children of our country are even worse: they watch more television than ever before and participate in fewer sports and other physical activities.

Lifestyle activity is designed to make you stop talking about getting off your duff and JUST DO IT! Simply defined, lifestyle activity is the extra motions and movements over and above what you would normally do in the course of a day. The calories burned from these extra activities are measured in small increments, but they add up. When you achieve your desired weight, the extra 150 calories burned through increased lifestyle activity may mean the difference between weight maintained or weight regained.

One of the best ways to assess how much activity you currently do each day is to wear a *pedometer*, a device that actually measures your steps. It is amazing how efficient we have become at combining our activities in order to reduce the number of our movements. For example, if there are stairs in the house, frequently a person will wait until there are more things to do upstairs before making the trip. Bad decision! See the following for further details.

Let's start with that marvelous invention, the car. Families are beginning to own as many cars as televisions. This means we don't walk anywhere. Added to that dismal fact is the new phenomenon of driving around for ten minutes looking for the parking space closest to the store. Now, you know you do that, at least sometimes. You say it's because you're in a hurry, but sometimes more time is wasted in driving around. What is also wasted is the opportunity to burn a few extra calories with a brisk walk from the rear of the parking lot. So, from now on, park where the people caring for their expensive new cars park. Your body and your car will thank you for it.

Bending and squatting. They don't sound like very glamorous activities, but the more you do, the more calories you burn. So clean up that spill with a cloth in your hand, not a mop. Bend down and pick up the paper, then drop it and pick it up again. Your flexibility will improve and the calories you burn will add up.

Climb those stairs. Do you wait for an elevator when you are only going to the next floor? Climbing stairs is a great calorie burner, and it's great for development of your leg muscles, too. Are you too out of shape to climb stairs? It isn't easy, but if you start with one flight a day and work your way up, eventually you'll be able to do ten flights at a time without overexerting yourself. Make a goal of walking up at least ten flights a day by the end of one month. Then see how many more flights you can add.

Do your own chores. Clean windows, vacuum floors, scrub floors on your knees. These are terrific activities to burn calories. Of course, if you already do these things, pat yourself on the back, then put more energy into each activity.

Fidget. You know, shake your foot, bounce your knee, tap your fingers, and so on. Studies have shown that all this extra movement burns extra calories. So, when you have to sit, don't sit still.

Move around while watching TV. Don't just sit there, iron your clothes. Do some extra picking up around the TV room. Make a point of moving during at least half of each program.

All of these activities added together should account for a better calorie burn each day. Add to this the fact that in being more active, your mental outlook will be healthier, too. What more could you ask from housework and stairs?

Day 21 Assignment: Write ten ideas to improve your lifestyle activity. Make sure that at least two situations can be implemented during your most difficult eating times. Implement the easiest idea today.

WORKSHEET

Ten Ideas to Improve My Lifestyle Activity:

1. _____

2. _____

3. _____

4. _____

5. _____

6. _____

7. _____

8. _____

9. _____

10. _____

Example:

1. Walk my child to school two days a week
2. Pick up stuff in the family room after dinner (my problem time)
3. Climb the steps at home at least three times between dinner and bedtime (my problem time)
4. Climb the stairs at work after lunch back to the office (four flights)
5. Wash my car every weekend
6. Do an extra household chore every weekend
7. Squat down when getting vegetables and fruit out of the bottom of the refrigerator
8. Walk from the back of the parking lot at the mall
9. Change the sheets on the bed an extra time per week
10. Reach for things in the back of cabinets

22

<hr>

Reward Systems

You have learned the importance of goal setting. Usually, the pride and satisfaction of achieving goals is sufficient to reinforce the new behavior. Sometimes, however, that feeling of gratification is not enough. Behavior is most often repeated when it is intermittently reinforced. This means that sometimes you get a reward for doing something and sometimes you don't get rewarded. While this works fine for mice in experiments, it is impractical for most people. Therefore, it is essential to develop your own reward system for some of the tougher behavioral changes.

If you are like most people, you may have immediately thought of food as a reward. *Wrong!* Food is not a reward. In its pure sense, food is the fuel with which we nourish our bodies. In other words, "eat to live," not "live to eat." This may be fairly unrealistic for some people, but food definitely should not used as a reward.

It is believed that using food treats to reward children's behavior eventually leads to obesity, because these children learn to seek food for comfort and reinforcement. Rewards, however, can be any one of a number of delightful, nonedible treats.

In determining how to set up a reward system, you must first consider which behavior to reward. It should be a specific goal but one that poses somewhat of a challenge. That is not to say that the other, easier goals you are working on should go by the wayside, but your primary focus at this time should be on the behavior that you have chosen to reward. In the meantime, reinforce your other positive behavioral changes by saying nice things to yourself. This is very important, not only for your mental attitude but because reinforcement of these other goals will keep you from ignoring them while you work on the tougher ones.

When deciding what the reward should be, select something that you would not obtain otherwise. In other words, don't select flowers for the dining-room table if you buy them every couple of weeks anyway.

A reward can be an object or an action. It can be new earrings, a new plant for the house, or the camera you always wanted. It can be making an extra long-distance phone call, having two hours of sheer laziness, or getting a facial. With some people, time is more precious than objects.

Rewards, like goals, should start small and increase in value as the difficulty of achieving the goals increases.

Then you can plan an every-three-month "ultimate" reward.

If this seems somewhat silly, consider the following: If someone told you that he would give you a million dollars to change a behavior, do you think you could do it, no matter how hard it seemed? Probably. Now, if the same person told you that he would give you a dollar to change that same behavior, do you think you would even try? Probably not. In other words, a reward is a reward only if you perceive it to be of great value. And we make changes only if we can find the proper motivation.

Now that you've been given some details as to how to do this, let's look at an example of exactly how rewards can be used.

Nancy is a thirty-seven-year-old account executive. She has gained 25 pounds over the past five years. She is ready to do something positive about her weight and has already started to make some positive changes in exercise and other behaviors.

Nancy's most difficult eating problem revolves around the office. She works for one of those companies where there is an endless supply of food. There are doughnuts and bagels almost every morning; there are crackers, cookies, microwave popcorn that smells heavenly, and candy out in the open all the time. Too, there is at least one monthly birthday celebration complete with cake.

Nancy has not exhibited any control over these foods as of late. She eats a doughnut or bagel with cream cheese every morning. Then she proceeds to munch her way through the rest of the day. Eating these foods is primarily a stress reliever, but her habits are so ingrained that even during days of minimal stress, she continues to nibble.

Nancy needs to attack this as three separate problems. First there is breakfast, then there are the snacks, and last are the special occasions, like parties and luncheons.

Breakfast is a difficult problem but not as difficult as the uncontrolled snacking during the day. Therefore, there are better boundaries on the breakfast issue. Nancy will make a plan to begin eating breakfast at home two mornings a week. On those mornings, she will not have any of the breakfast treats at work. On the other three mornings, she will cut her usual portion in half, and supplement each with a small glass of skim milk. She should expect to accomplish this goal half of the time initially and 75 percent of the time after two weeks. As a reward for attaining this goal, Nancy wants to buy a better pair of walking shoes. She has been walking daily and her shoes are adequate, but she wants a better pair.

After the second week, Nancy will increase having breakfast at home to four days a week, with the same plan for the other days at work. This goal will be worked on for another two weeks. At this point there is a new necklace for Nancy to match a dress for which she doesn't have the right accessories. She gets the necklace if she accomplishes the goal seven of the eight days in the two-week period.

Finally, in the fifth week, Nancy must decide whether or not she wants to continue to eat a bagel or doughnut one day a week for breakfast at the office. She chooses to do so. Although she knows it's not the healthiest breakfast, she also knows she is not a great "morning person." So, on the days when she is running late and misses breakfast at home, she will still have the option of breakfast at work. And that's a big improvement over her current behavior.

For her continuing adherence to her breakfast goal, Nancy will reward herself at one-month and two-month intervals. After that point, the rewards will end and she will monitor her behavior on a periodic monitoring form (see chapter 30).

Nancy will do similar reinforcements with changing behaviors for munching on special occasions. She will take on only one major change at a time.

It takes a great deal of mental effort to devise and implement a reward system. But the "rewards" in terms of the behavior outcomes are worth it.

Day 22 Assignment: Now is the time to pick one of your more difficult goals. It must be one that you've wanted to accomplish but haven't been able to thus far. It must be a very specific goal, such that you can measure your success in achieving it. Using the form provided, write up a set of rewards of increasing value as you accomplish this goal and continue to repeat and/or improve it.

WORKSHEET

Reward System

My goal: _____

_____

_____

_____

How I expect to accomplish it in increments: _____

_____

_____

_____

What my reward will be at each increment: _____

_____

_____

_____

_____

Example:

My goal: To start bringing my lunch to work. This has been a problem because I rush around in the morning and either forget to take the things I need or don't have the time to gather the things together.

How I expect to accomplish it in increments: First, make a plan. I will gather the items I need the night before so that there is less rushing in the morning. I will first make a goal of bringing my lunch three days a week for the first two weeks. Then I will increase it to four days a week thereafter and will even try for all five days, but will be satisfied if I meet the goal of four days per week.

What my reward will be at each increment: At the end of the first week, if I have met the three-day goal, I will reward myself by buying a pair of earrings to match an outfit that I have. At the end of the second week, when I have met my goal of bringing my lunch three days a week for both weeks, I will make a long-distance phone call to a friend to whom I usually write. At the end of the fourth week, if I've been bringing my lunch four days a week for the prior two weeks, I'll give myself the "grand reward," which will be a new exercise outfit. This is a bit frivolous, but it will reward both my lunch behavior and my exercise behavior.

23

Just My Imagination

D o you have a powerful imagination? You need one, or to develop one, if you are to achieve permanent changes in your eating habits.

There are two ways that your imagination can work for you. It can be used to deter you from your problem food, or it can be used to steer you in a better direction.

First, the deterrent visualization. This is done when you anticipate eating a food that you don't really want but are tempted to eat anyway.

If the tempting food is an ice cream sundae, for example, you can use your imagination to work for you in the following way:

Close your eyes. Visualize the ice cream sundae as you normally see it. Imagine every detail. There is the ice cream, maybe marshmallow chocolate chip. Then there is the hot fudge, which, when poured on, begins to melt the ice cream. Whipped cream delicately swirled on the top makes a delectable design. Chopped nuts lie delicately on the whipped cream, providing the irresistible crunch. And then there's my favorite, the maraschino cherry on top, with a bit of its light red juice trickling down the whipped cream.

Did that make you hungry? If not, visualize your own concoction that brings a smile to your face and gets you salivating.

Now, let's look at the sundae again. This time, it has been sitting on the kitchen counter for three days. It has melted and flowed over the parfait glass and onto the counter. The puddle on the counter is sticky with dried ice cream in the areas where only a thin layer reached. Then there are areas on the counter where there are blobs of fuzzy-looking white stuff—what was once the whipped cream. In the parfait glass itself is a pool of melted, warm ice cream, whipped cream, and hot fudge. It is just a blob of mostly brown stuff, but there is a touch of something greenish, too. The cherry is dried and cracked. And of course, there is that aroma. . . .

So, how does that sundae sound now? If that method helps, use it whenever you are faced with a tempting item that you really want to avoid.

If that method is not the answer for you, there is an alternative. It deals with the positive side of your visualization and reinforces your behavior.

First, you visualize a situation during which you have trouble controlling your eating. You imagine specific decisions and your successful adherence to each decision. The following is an example:

Restaurant eating with friends frequently turns into an eating orgy. There are too many temptations and the casual atmosphere makes clear thinking more difficult.

This is where imagination works especially well. It enables you to decide in advance how to handle the difficult decisions. This works much better than just thinking, "I'll try to be good," because spontaneous decisions are dangerous. Premeditated decisions are much easier.

Your imagination works best when you have had some prior experience with the situation. In this example, the restaurant is familiar to you. Start at the beginning. Picture yourself arriving at the restaurant. See the restaurant in full detail in your mind—the layout, the people, everything. When you arrive there you usually wait for a table to become available. You are escorted to the bar. See yourself with your friends being seated at the bar. Here's the first decision to make. Will you have a drink or just club soda? Decide and write down that decision. Oh no, there's popcorn on the table. Visualize yourself ignoring it, not even looking at it.

Now imagine your table is ready. Imagine your group being shown to the table. How does the table look? Are there flowers on the table? If so, try to sit nearer to them so that there is less room in front of you for foods to be placed. Are there crackers or bread on the table? If so, move them away from you. Decide whether you will eat any bread with the dinner or forgo it for a shared portion of dessert later.

The waiter is now coming to take your order. You have called the restaurant in advance to find out what kinds of foods are available. You have made a decision of an entrée that you will enjoy and that can be prepared in a healthful fashion. There is no reason to go to a restaurant and eat something you dislike. Hopefully, there are many dishes from which you can choose that are both healthful and tasty. See yourself ordering a prechosen entrée and specifying how you want it prepared. You order salad with dressing on the side. You skip the appetizer but agree to share dessert with your friend.

See yourself eating very slowly. Go to the restaurant armed with first-rate conversation. He who talks a lot does not have as much time to eat. Drink at least two glasses of water during the meal—it will fill you up and provide pauses in your eating. Put your fork down between bites. Blot your mouth with your napkin after every two bites. All these details take concentration, and when that happens, you focus less on consuming every bite. This is how thin people eat naturally, without thinking about it.

When you still have at least three bites of food left on your plate, put down your napkin just next to your plate and place your silverware on the plate with the fork tines down. This will indicate to the waiter that you are finished with your meal. Then, even if you were tempted to eat what was left, you would be too embarrassed to start eating again. Your waiter will take your plate and the temptation will be gone. Remember, these are all things that you are visualizing before you get to the restaurant.

When deciding on dessert, take into account how strict you've already been and what your decision should be about dessert. If you decide to share dessert with the others, you'll obviously eat less and feel very powerful about your control.

Most important, visualize yourself leaving the restaurant having been successful at every juncture. You made each decision that needed to be made ahead of time, and you stuck with those decisions. Doesn't that feel wonderful? Now go out and do it in reality. It won't be half as hard as you thought it would.

One addendum to this approach. There are times that we intentionally go out and "blow it." While this need not happen too often, as long as you have decided to do it, don't attempt to make decisions to control your eating if you don't intend to stick with them. That would make you feel like a total failure.

Day 23 Assignment: Think of a dangerous situation that is coming up in the near future that involves eating. Use your powers of visualization and imagination to make decisions in advance and see yourself as successful at various junctures. On the sheet provided, record the specific decisions you make and picture your success each day until the event occurs. Then reward yourself if you were 90 percent successful in accomplishing your intentions.

WORKSHEET

The upcoming event is: _____

_____

_____

_____

The specific decisions are: _____

_____

_____

If I am 90% successful, I will reward myself with: _____

_____

_____

_____

_____

Example:

The upcoming event is: A cookout at my friend's house. This is tough because I love all the food at this type of event—hot dogs, hamburgers, potato chips, potato salad, macaroni salad, et cetera.

The specific decisions are:
1. I will have an Alba Milkshake before I leave for the cookout.
2. I will skip the potato chips because I would not be able to control the portion.
3. I will have one mayonnaise-based salad in approximately a half-cup portion.

4. I will have one hamburger without cheese and half of one hot dog.

5. I will have two serving-spoons full of baked beans.

6. I will drink only calorie-free beverages.

If I am 90% successful, I will reward myself with: A pedicure, the next day.

24

Thirty Behavioral
Improvements

*O*kay, you want the specifics of improving your
behavior? Here they are.
    **GET THE TEMPTATION FOODS OUT OF
THE HOUSE.** Do you use the excuse that you must have
goodies around the house for your family or for unexpected
company? This is unnecessary and provides you with un-
wanted temptation. There must be some foods that you
can have on hand for these people that provide less of a
temptation for you. Besides, if the tempting food is junk-
type stuff, they don't need it either. Do you tell yourself
that you'll just have to learn to resist all these things being
around? You say that everyone shouldn't have to suffer
just because you're watching your weight? Again, initially
it is not a good idea to test your control too much. Remember abstinence versus control? Initially abstinence is
better with some foods, until your confidence grows. Get
the very tempting foods out of the house for a month.

Then, as you gradually replace some of them, monitor how you deal with them and decide which ones may be there only on an occasional basis.

DO NOT BUY DIET FOODS. This does not mean that everything labeled "diet" is bad. A diet soda is okay and so are the low-fat frozen chocolate bars. But if you are in the habit of purchasing diet foods that do not have sugar or fat but still have calories, and then you proceed to eat hefty quantities of these foods, that is not good. Remember that even if a product has minimal calories, it is a bad habit to nibble on foods in an unconscious manner.

PORTION ANY SMALL-SIZED FOODS. Did you ever notice that small foods are dangerous? Our ability to eat them in an unconscious manner is greater than with other foods. Think of snack foods. Whether sweets, nuts, chips, or crackers, small things usually end up as our snack-attack foods. Even cereal can be harmful. I once went from eating sweets as a snack to eating lightly sweetened dry cereal. What could be the harm? I thought. There was no fat in the cereal. The problem was, I would buy a 16-ounce box of cereal at noon one day and grab handfuls of it whenever I felt like it. In a matter of forty-eight hours, the cereal would be gone. A 16-ounce box of cereal has 1,760 calories in it. Therefore, I was eating 880 extra calories per day! That's terrible, especially since I never thought I was doing anything wrong. Bite-size foods are difficult to eliminate because we are less aware of our eating them. But all you need to do is portion the serving you desire, or know you should eat, and when that's gone, you're finished eating that food.

WRITE A SNACK PLAN. Writing a snack plan takes the spontaneity out of snacking and puts the control back in. Initially, this is the best procedure. Then, when you are accustomed to having a variety of planned snacks, eating them in the right portions will come more naturally to you. And you won't have to do so much planning. Make sure to have snacks that you enjoy and that are filling. That way, when you deviate from the usual with a splurge, you won't dread going back to the usual options.

In the above example it would be easy to include cereal on a snack plan if the portion was accounted for and if the cereal was measured.

BUY GROCERIES FROM A LIST. Do you go to the grocery store and wander up and down each aisle? That frequently leads to picking up items that you would not normally purchase. Make sure you do not go to the grocery store when you are hungry. Food does not look so tempting when you are not starving.

DO NOT SERVE FAMILY-STYLE. This common practice among families leads to extra helpings when the person isn't even hungry. Here's the scenario:

You're sitting at the table having spaghetti. The salad has been eaten. Your spaghetti has been eaten. You are not stuffed, but you are not hungry, either. But here's this platter of spaghetti right in front of you, and as you are talking to the others at the table, you take an extra helping. *Bang!* An extra few hundred calories you could have skipped or at least saved for later. Portion all foods in the kitchen. Bring the plate with the specified quantity to the table.

GET OUT OF THE HOUSE AT THE TROUBLE TIMES. For many of us, our most difficult eating time is difficult only when we are at home. It is the boredom or the television that most frequently gets us into trouble, not the time itself. So, get out more often. This is an excellent time to do more exercise or lifestyle activities.

TAKE SNACKS TO WORK. If you have trouble controlling yourself at work, or if you get hungry at work and don't have anything to eat, take suitable snacks with you. Know that you will get hungry and be prepared to take care of that hunger. Going four or five hours without eating is too long.

LIMIT TELEVISION WATCHING. There is a direct correlation between television watching and weight gain. If you are a victim of TV nibbling, watch less TV. Do more exercise and lifestyle activities.

ENGAGE IN ACTIVITIES THAT PRECLUDE EATING. Getting out of the house helps to control eating. Keeping your hands and mind occupied when at home helps, too. Helpful activities include sewing, knitting, writing, playing the piano, even showering—anything that means you can't eat simultaneously.

HAVE FAMILY MEMBERS GET THEIR OWN SNACKS. Do you nibble while handing out snacks to the kids? Do you get up and get your spouse's ice cream? *Stop it!* Unless you have very small children, you need not be the one who hands out the goodies. If you must, at least portion them out when you are not hungry.

GO TO FEWER SOCIAL EATING FUNCTIONS

DURING LOW-CONTROL PERIODS. This is not to suggest that you give up your social life. But when you are not doing well at controlling your eating habits, you don't want to subject yourself to undue temptation. That is, unless you are better at eating out than eating at home. In that case, go to as many social eating functions as you possibly can.

EAT BEFORE YOU EAT. Don't forget the importance of this. Drink a large glass of water before each meal. Have a small snack before the meals at which you tend to eat large quantities.

WAIT TWENTY MINUTES BEFORE HAVING AN UNPLANNED SNACK. Play the waiting game. When you feel like eating but it hasn't been that long since you last ate, wait twenty minutes before you give in to the urge. In all likelihood, you will watch the clock for the first five minutes and then will forget about the desire to eat for at least thirty minutes. It almost always works that way.

PUT LEFTOVERS AWAY BEFORE SITTING DOWN TO A MEAL. As I already stated, you shouldn't serve family-style. There may still be a temptation to grab an extra spoonful of a leftover before it is covered and put in the refrigerator. Therefore, put away such items before you sit down to eat.

THINK OF THE HIGHEST-CALORIE FOOD ON THE PLATE AS THE DESSERT. When I first started eating spaghetti for dinner, I was in wonderful control. Then, as time went by, my portion control slipped a bit.

Finally, in an effort to do better, I would first focus on the salad and cooked vegetable and view my pasta as dessert. Guess what? It worked!

REARRANGE FOOD SUPPLIES. This is the old "out of sight, out of mind" trick and it really works. If you put the most tempting foods out of reach and out of view, you will forget they are there. This will happen even when you are rooting around for something to eat. If you do decide to eat the food that is out of reach and you have to get on a chair to reach it, there's a chance that you will feel foolish enough to stop yourself.

AVOID DISTRACTING ACTIVITIES WHEN EATING. Eating should be a pure activity. That means no television, no reading, and no working while eating. This may sound nearly impossible, but it's not. You lose your awareness of eating when you involve yourself in activities simultaneously while eating.

EAT EVERYTHING WITH A FORK. This sounds pretty unrealistic. But think about it. How many cookies can you eat with a fork? Or potato chips? This proves that bite-sized foods are troublesome. So, try to eat everything with a fork, and increase your awareness of what constitutes your diet.

PLAN A DELAY BETWEEN THE SALAD AND THE MEAL. This is how you eat in a restaurant. Do the same at home. Remember that it takes twenty minutes for your brain to get the message that your stomach has food in it. Delaying consumption after the first course will help your brain get the right message.

EAT MORE SLOWLY. I can't reiterate this enough. Most people admit that they eat too rapidly. Therefore, put down your fork between bites, drink a sip of water between bites, and time your meal to make it last twenty minutes. Think about this every time you eat.

LEAVE A SMALL AMOUNT OF FOOD ON YOUR PLATE. Were you forced to be a member of the clean-plate club? Do this no longer. Don't subject your children to this, either. Leave just one bite on the plate. The feeling of control this provides can't be beaten.

EAT AND SNACK AT REGULAR TIMES. Plan ahead, know when you need to eat, and bring food if necessary. Remember that when you leave eating to chance, you will probably make a poor decision.

COMPENSATE FOR HEAVIER EATING TIMES. When you have a party or special occasion or just end up eating more than usual on a given day, eat a bit less the following day. This will quickly restore your feeling of control.

DO NOT EAT FOODS YOU DON'T LIKE. This sounds like easy advice to follow, but when people diet, they frequently feel that they must suffer to lose weight. Part of that suffering includes eating food they don't like. So, don't ever waste calories on foods you don't like. There are plenty of foods you can incorporate into your daily menu without blowing your control because you like them too much.

HIGH-CALORIE FOODS SHOULD REQUIRE EXTRA PREPARATION. These foods should not be so easy that you just open a box and eat. Extra preparation gives you extra time to think about eating and make sure it is what you really want to do.

EAT ON SMALLER PLATES. This will make it look like there is more food than there really is. Remember, it's important to please your mental appetite as well as your physical appetite.

PLAN FOR A CERTAIN NUMBER OF FAVORITE FOODS. Making a list of forever-forbidden foods will ultimately lead you to cheat. Plan to have your favorite foods occasionally, when you can truly enjoy them.

DON'T EAT IN THE CAR. Eating in the car does not allow you to give your full attention to what you are eating. You will feel as if you haven't eaten because you have not mentally focused on enjoying your food. You will also drive more safely if you use all of your mind and both of your hands.

SIT DOWN TO EAT. If you are a taster during the cooking process, you could be picking up an extra 200 calories per day. That's 1 pound every seventeen days! If you need to test the food, portion a small amount, then sit down to taste it. That will stop you from constant tasting.

The above should keep you busy for at least another thirty days. If you really work on them one at a time, some of the suggestions could take a month all by themselves. The slower this process is, the more likely it is that you will maintain your behavioral changes.

Day 24 Assignment: In the past twenty-three days, you have made many changes. Make a list of the top ten new behaviors that make you feel proud of yourself. These should be the behaviors that you do consistently and feel confident that you will continue to do, no matter what. This activity will go a long way toward making you feel that you have gained a great deal of control over your eating behavior.

WORKSHEET

The Top Ten Behaviors I am Doing Consistently

1. _____
2. _____
3. _____
4. _____
5. _____
6. _____
7. _____
8. _____
9. _____
10. _____

Example:

1. I am exercising aerobically at least three days every week.

2. I am eating more than 500 calories by 3:00 P.M. each day.

3. I am eating nonfat frozen yogurt in place of ice cream.

4. I am eating two vegetarian meals each week for dinner.

5. I am eating fish at least twice each week.

6. I am climbing at least four flights of stairs each day.

7. I am parking farther away at the mall than I used to.

8. I have increased my fiber intake to 10 grams per day.

9. I am planning my evening snacks.

10. I am eating a snack before a dangerous dinner at least once a week.

25

Taking Failure
in Stride

A s previously stated, this is not really a diet book as
such. It is intended to help you gain control of your
eating habits and thereby lose weight. I have repeatedly tried to discourage the black-and-white approach
to eating, insisting that it only ensures failure. You cannot
look at eating as either bingeing or starving. You must
learn to live in the gray zone, and in doing so you will
have good days and bad days. There will be times when
you are very pleased with your food selections and days
when you are disgusted with those selections. Why this
happens is not important; just know that it will happen.
You will not be perfect, nor will you strive for perfection.
This should not be depressing. Even thin people have bad
eating days, but it does not concern them as much. They
do not exaggerate the problem in their minds, and you
should strive to emulate their attitude.

How you prevent one or two bad days from becoming

a total downfall is what's important. This chapter will deal specifically with how to prevent you from letting one failure ruin your well-laid plans.

The most important thing you must do at this point is begin to examine what behaviors you have changed that you feel certain you can sustain. These changes will constitute your *foundation*.

A foundation is the basis upon which you build your other attempts at improving your eating habits. Sometimes these attempts will be positive. Other times the attempts that you have built will crumble down to the foundation. The point is that the foundation will not crack, no matter how bad other eating habits get. For example, remember the importance of exercise and how it should be independent of your eating habits. This means you should think of it like brushing your teeth. You do this every day, regardless of how you eat. Therefore, you must always exercise, regardless of how you eat.

Other suggestions for your foundation include basing it on increasing your water intake, eating breakfast, planning 2-2-2-1 dinners, always serving a cooked vegetable at dinner, not eating anything after 8:00 P.M., keeping a snack diary, weighing yourself at least every week, and reporting your weight to a friend every week. Choose four of these or other suggestions from the book and build your foundation today.

Another essential for keeping a bad day of eating from turning into a downfall is to refuse to accept the idea that since you have failed you might as well get it all out of your system. We have already seen that this is a bad idea for two reasons. First, it ignores the fact that whatever the bad eating that occurred, you have to burn off those calories as well as all the additional calories you add to them. This also implies that you've been depriving yourself of many foods that you feel are forbidden. That is why there is this need to binge on all of them before getting back to what you perceive as "perfection eating." Secondly, you assume that you can get back on track. We now know that the guilt over bingeing is very strong, making a fresh start extremely difficult.

If you can identify situations ahead of time that may cause a downfall, you can develop coping strategies. Have a plan of attack for the identified and the unexpected occasions that cause problems with your eating habits. For example, the winter holidays usually mean a weight gain of 10 or more pounds over a two-month period. How are you going to handle it this year?

First, you will focus on your foundation. Next, you will do a lot of writing of plans for snacks, parties, eating at work, and so on. You will increase your exercise (at a time when you would be more likely to decrease it) in order to compensate for some of the excess calories. You will allow a splurge meal for the actual holiday dates themselves and one more splurge meal each week. But you will make plans for the extra meal each week so that it is not without some level of control.

Under these circumstances, you are unlikely to completly lose sight of your goals. You'll get back on track faster. Soon you'll be eating like a person who never had a control problem, much to your surprise.

Day 25 Assignment: Decide what your foundation will be for the next several months. This should be at least four fundamental behaviors that are moderately challenging.

WORKSHEET

Foundation

1. _____

2. _____

3. _____

4. _____

Example:

1. I will weigh myself and record it at least once a week and no more frequently than once a day.

2. I will exercise aerobically at least three days each week.

3. I will drink at least 64 ounces of water each day.

4. I will continue to write goals for my eating behavior on a weekly basis.

26

The Waiting Game

You are reading this book not because your primary problem is eating too much at meals. If anything, you claim to be in great control at meals and can even skip most of them if you wanted to. But you start snacking around 4:00 P.M. and don't stop until you go to bed around 11:00 P.M. It's those darn snack attacks.

Because of this, you must learn the rules of the waiting game, and then learn to win. The waiting game is the primary key to conquering snacking habits. It provides you with control in situations that usually seem uncontrollable.

The waiting game is based on one simple principle with several variations. Its basis is always to wait twenty minutes before having an unplanned snack. Whether that sounds easy or very difficult, it is extremely important.

Studies have shown that overweight people·eat by the clock and other external stimuli. If you were to place overweight people and normal-weight people in a room where they didn't know what time it is, and then place them in a room where they think it is noon by a clock on the wall when it is actually only 10:00 A.M., the normal-weight group will go on with their activities, with no notice of the clock and/or its relation to their appetite. The overweight group will complain of hunger because they perceive that it is time to eat.

Therefore, it stands to reason that if overweight people are more attentive to external cues in relation to their appetite, they can use these cues to help control their eating.

Playing the waiting game also means eating more slowly. When you take in food too quickly you go from a feeling of being starved to a stuffed feeling without ever having felt just satisfied. This is because your brain doesn't received the signal telling it that your stomach is full.

It's difficult not to wolf down the foods we most enjoy. They taste so good that we just can't seem to wait for the next bite. But you must remember one thing: It's only good while it's in your mouth! Seriously. Your taste buds are on your tongue. When you eat quickly, you are swallowing one bite while reaching for another. Once the food is going down your throat, you've lost the ability to taste it. So, chew slowly. Savor each bite. Make it last longer in your mouth.

In learning to eat slowly, it is helpful to watch people who are naturally thin. This observation works best at dinner in a restaurant. Watch how they take great pains to get their napkin situated properly. See them drink a lot of water. When their salad comes, they make sure there is just the right amount of dressing, not too much, not too little. When the meal comes, they take a great deal of time making sure they are prepared to eat it. They readjust their napkin. They drink more water, they adjust the plate. Then, when they finally start to eat, they play with the food. They move it around the plate. They blot their mouths between bites. They talk, sometimes incessantly, and since they can't eat while they are talking, they finish only half of what they were served. Then the waiter comes to take one of the fast-eaters' plates and the thin person tells him to take his plate, too. It's wonderfully disgusting to watch these people in action. Strive your hardest to eat just as they do.

Day 26 Assignment: The next time you want to have an unplanned snack, wait twenty minutes. Right now, write down specifics of when the unplanned snacking is the hardest to resist. What have you done when you have been the most successful in getting it under control? Put these elements into your waiting plan.

WORKSHEET

The times that uncontrolled snacking is still the most difficult: _____

_____

_____

_____

What I have done to make these times more successful:

_____

_____

How I will incorporate these successes into my goals:____

_____

_____

_____

Example:

The times that uncontrolled snacking is still the most difficult: After dinner is still the toughest time. I still crave sweets, but less than I used to. Before dinner is still a somewhat difficult time. I am tired then and my resistance is low.

What I have done to make these times more successful:
After dinner, I:
Plan my snacks
Watch less television

Have a lower-sugar, low-fat snack in place of my former sweets

Do lifestyle activity during the evening

Before dinner I:

Exercise at least three times a week when I first get off from work

Eat a snack before I leave the office so that I'm not starving when I get home

Drink a large glass of water when I first get home

How I will incorporate these successes into my goals:

I will continue to plan my snacks.

I will continue to watch less television.

I am working on developing a goal not to snack while watching television, but I'm not quite ready.

I will continue to push the water—this helps.

27

Restaurant and Other Social Eating

I believe eating out is one of the most difficult situations encountered by people who are trying to control their eating habits. Chances are, you consider eating out a special occasion and therefore tend to make related excuses as to why you do not stay in good control in these situations. The problem with that thinking is that Americans now eat 50 percent or more of their meals away from home. Furthermore, on the average, we eat in (or get take-out from) fast-food restaurants at least one or more times a week.

There are numerous problems with eating out, beginning with what I mentioned above. Eating out is considered a special occasion. This is despite the fact that the frequency of eating out is high and therefore less effort is made to control consumption. A person might say, "I'll try to be good," but that's not nearly specific enough to ensure any degree of success. And despite what someone says, her true intentions may not really be good.

Another problem with eating out is that the meal most frequently is dinner, which occurs at the most difficult time of the day to control eating. It is also the time when the calories are needed the least.

There are two primary problems with eating in restaurants. The first is that the temptations are greater. We do things in restaurants that we would not do at home. You probably do not serve bread with your dinner at home except when entertaining. Bread, however, is likely the first item you reach for in a restaurant. You may even consider the bread you eat in a restaurant to be your number-one downfall.

Another temptation in restaurants is dessert. While you may ultimately eat sweets at some time after dinner, you are probably not in the habit of eating formal desserts at home. In a restaurant, though, your favorite dishes are already prepared.

The second problem with restaurant eating is that even when you have conquered the temptations, the food is not prepared the same way as you would make it at home. Most of us are trying to cook more healthfully at home. We use less oils, eat more vegetables, and avoid sauces. Eating healthful foods in restaurants is difficult to achieve at best. The food is frequently cooked with a great deal of fat, and there is more fat, in the form of sauce, added over the entrées. Often vegetables are not available except in salads. When you ask for food to be prepared in a special way, often the restaurant can't or won't do it.

Therefore, your choices lack variety because there are so few safe selections. Lack of variety leads to beginning to indulge in your old favorites. Then, restaurants are as dangerous as they were before you began this process.

Remember, even if you stay in pretty good control at dinner, the urge to nibble later at night will still present a challenge, because that desire has little to do with hunger and everything to do with habit. Therefore, to help the evening snacking from being too damaging, try to keep dinners light! That is very hard to do when eating out. That's the bad news. The good news is that this chapter will give you suggestions on how to make your best possible choices.

The two most important factors to control in a restaurant are fat and total calories. This can be done in various ways depending on the restaurant. The first thing to keep in mind is what this book has taught you so far. Think about the chapter on fat. Think about the importance of controlling your portions when dining out.

Remember to *eat before you eat*. The last thing you want to do is arrive at a restaurant hungry. This can be difficult because most of us desire to eat what we have paid for, even if the portion is large. Do remember that no matter what route you take to control your restaurant eating, "doggie bags" are no longer considered gauche. So, if it is worth eating, it's worth eating twice.

Following is a list of suggestions that should facilitate your dining experience. Use it as a guide. When it doesn't work in a particular situation, eat half of the item and skip the obviously dangerous foods.

In general, remember that the greatest source of fat we consume is in the animal products we eat. A 3-ounce portion is advisable for an entrée. That is equivalent to the size of a deck of cards. Restaurants generally serve two to five times that much. Try to follow these guidelines when ordering:

Entrées

1. "Wine broiled" or "dry broiled" white fish such as sole or flounder are your best choices. Be sure to specify *no fat*. Do not say "no butter." If they use margarine, they'll still use it and you don't want that.
2. A shrimp cocktail or plain steamed shellfish as an entrée is a lean choice.
3. If you are going to eat chicken, try to get a broiled breast cutlet that is prepared without the skin. If this is not available, order plain chicken with sauce on the side. Then meticulously take off all the skin and fat.
4. Veal and lamb chops are generally fatty choices, but if you cut off the fat and keep the portion small, they can work.
5. Your best choice for beef is a small filet mignon.

Side Dishes

1. In an Italian restaurant, order pasta with marinara sauce on the side.
2. In a Chinese restaurant, order white (not fried) rice.

3. In any other restaurant, order a plain baked potato —it's the only safe choice. Rice or pasta frequently have fat added to them. A baked potato comes to you plain, and you bring your nonfat powder to sprinkle on the potato.
4. Order a green vegetable in addition to the starch. It will give you one more safe thing to fill up on.

Appetizers

1. Eliminate rolls, or limit them and compensate by cutting back on something else. Avoid butter and margarine.
2. Have as large a tossed salad as possible. Bring your own nonfat salad dressing or order dressing on the side and dip your fork in the dressing before you stab your lettuce. Request fresh vegetables in the salad and avoid croutons, cheese, egg yolks, olives, bacon bits, and mayonnaise-based items.
3. Avoid soups—they are usually high in sodium and fat. If the restaurant prepares prime rib, they may cut the fat off and throw it into the soup crock, even if it's vegetable soup.

Desserts

1. Fresh berries are an excellent choice.
2. Skip dessert at the restaurant and go out to a frozen-yogurt place later and order a 5-ounce cup of nonfat yogurt.

3. Have *one* bite of a rich dessert, but don't be the first to pass it around or you'll end up finishing it.

The following are safer selections at various types of restaurants:

Chinese

1. Order a bowl of wonton soup and eat half the wontons.
2. Order entrées that are steamed, not stir-fried. For example: moo goo gai pan, chow mein, and chop suey.
3. Avoid the dried noodles on the table (they are fried).
4. Order white rice instead of fried rice.
5. Have *one* fortune cookie for dessert.

Italian

1. Spaghetti marinara or pasta with red clam sauce are ideal choices.
2. Most veal dishes are breaded and fried.
3. Chicken cacciatore is sometimes a safe choice, especially if a skinless chicken breast is used.

Mexican

1. Large salads are good, but a taco salad is among the highest fat and calorie items you could eat in any restaurant. This is due to the guacamole, sour cream, cheese, refried beans, and fried tortilla.

2. Flour tortillas are generally low in fat. A chicken fajita, with lots of lettuce, tomato, and salsa, is a good bet.

Social events such as parties and weddings can have a devastating effect on your control. Many of these occasions are even more difficult than restaurant eating because they make use of help-yourself buffets—an uncontrolled-eater's nightmare.

The same rules apply as far as avoiding fatty foods, watching portions of animal products, and filling up on low-calorie bulky foods before going. In addition, there are a few more behavioral techniques that might help.

The first is to wear something tight. That may sound strange, but the less room your stomach has to expand in your clothes, the less you will be able to eat. Of course, if you don't eat slowly under these circumstances, you will suddenly bloat out and feel like you are ready to explode.

Another trick to employ at the buffet table is to survey all the foods before taking a single bite. This will allow you to make your calories count. Why fill up on wasted calories when you can savor a few delicious calories of a favorite food?

Stand or sit away from the food. This is the "out of sight, out of mind" principle. If you are not staring at the food, you will not eat as much of it.

Interchange alcoholic drinks with club soda. This will cut down your alcohol calories while still allowing you a small indulgence.

Compensate the day before and the day after. You should never starve before going to a party, because you'll end up eating the equivalent of all the missed meals in one hour of party eating. Simply eat lighter the day before and the day after, and you'll have a bit more leeway.

The most important aspect of social eating is the fact that it is social. Learning to focus on the friends, the family, and the business environment will help take some of the emphasis off the meal itself. Doing the right tricks and techniques will eventually allow the right focus to happen with less forethought.

Day 27 Assignment: Determine the percentage of time you eat meals away from home. Then determine the percentage of time the meals that are eaten out create challenges. Make a written plan to make choices easier in half of those situations. See examples on the form below.

WORKSHEET

The percentage of time I eat meals away from home: ___

_____

_____

The percentage of time that these meals pose an eating challenge: _____

_____

_____

How I will reduce these difficult times by 50 percent: ___

_____

_____

Example:

The percentage of time I eat meals away from home: 57 percent. This includes eating the following meals out: five lunches, 1 breakfast, 3 dinners.

The percentage of time that these meals pose an eating challenge: 67 percent (6 out of 9) of these meals still present a problem. This includes the three dinners, one breakfast, and two of the lunches (because I still bring my lunch only two days a week).

How I will reduce these difficult times by 50 percent:
1. I will start bringing my lunch all five days a week. I've been doing well at being better organized and it should not be a problem. That takes care of two days.
2. I will start going to a Chinese restaurant for one of the three dinners each week. I have good control when eating there. That takes care of one more meal.

3. The above two meet my stated objective, but I will try to make an improvement in the way I handle dinner one more night each week.

28

~~~~~~~~~~

Support Mechanisms

O	*vereating* is a common problem, but the people affected by it are a diverse group. Most are basically ashamed by their lack of control over their eating habits, which makes getting help a difficult step. That is a fact despite the billions of dollars spent each year on weight-loss centers and diet programs. It is still a private agony for most people.

This makes deciding on whether to include a friend or loved one in your exercise and weight-loss program an even more difficult decision, but one that must be made. The idea of including a partner in your program is based on the acknowledgment that the quest to control your eating behavior is an ongoing process. If you're lucky, you'll work on it for a lifetime. There is no terminal point where this all becomes second nature; significantly easier, yes, but not second nature. Therefore, a partner can serve to reinforce and to add balance to your approach to this. Partnerships usually are not temporary situations. They are long-term investments, thereby reinforcing your long-term commitment to changing your eating and exercise habits for life.

There are advantages and disadvantages to including a partner in your eating program. If you don't know how a partner could help you in your goals, you need to learn what such a partnership is: It is an agreement between you and someone else to help you stay on track with your eating goals. To select this person you must take into account many factors. One of the ideal characteristics of the person you select is that he or she be trying in a similar fashion to learn how to control his or her eating habits.

The advantages of having a partner include the fact that this person is in the same situation as you in terms of trying to achieve the same goals. He therefore has more compassion and understanding in regard to the difficulties. Another advantage to having a partner is that he will have current, resourceful ideas on how to keep making this work. It's the "two heads are better than one" theory. You can serve as a reinforcer of your partner's behavior as well, although this is not necessary.

A partner in exercise can be a definite advantage. When you arrange to meet at a specific time for a walk or other type of workout, you will not be as tempted to skip out at the last minute. You will not want to disappoint her because she arranged to meet you. She is counting on you.

There are some times when a partner is not a good idea. If you decide to include someone on a frequent basis to share some intimate problems with eating, you must be prepared to deal with some criticism or other form of correction on occasion. That is the purpose of a partner. He is supposed to help get you back on track and keep you on track as long as possible.

Another problem is that if this person starts to fail in his attempts to control his eating, you must be prepared to go on without him if your encouragement is not sufficient to help him. You cannot allow yourself to fail because your partner has failed.

The disadvantage to having a partner in an exercise program is that the two individuals must be fairly evenly matched physically. If you are walking with someone and must slow down for him to keep up with you, the exercise is not doing you any good. Unless you were doing side-by-side exercise, such as stationary bicycling, the two of you must be performing at an equal pace.

To determine whether a partner is right for you, first set some ground rules. Following are examples that should help:

1. A partner is not in competition with you. You are not in a race to get this done fast. It is a slow process.
2. A partner will help you with a problem at any hour of the day or night. This is important so that you feel you can count on this person to help you solve problems anytime.
3. A partner will do what she thinks is best to help you get back on track if she feels you have deviated too far from your course.

4. A partner is knowledgeable about what you are trying to accomplish.
5. A partner will not make decisions for you.
6. A partner will not betray your confidence or embarrass you in front of other people.

If you set these and other guidelines, it will help you to decide whether partnership is right for you and if you know someone who could fill that role for you. You can decide if a partner is appropriate for exercise alone or in addition to the eating behavior.

Day 28 Assignment: Decide if a partner is appropriate for you to exercise with two times of your 5 times per week schedule. Make a determination if you have a friend or someone else who can be your eating behavior partner on a long-term basis.

WORKSHEET

Should I have an exercise partner two of five days per week? _____

_____

_____

Is there someone who can be a long-term eating-behavior partner? _____
_____
_____

How will I use that person to accomplish my long-term goals? _____
_____
_____

Example:

Should I have an exercise partner two of five days per week? Yes. Since I go to a gym two days a week, I can go with my friend. This will be helpful because we can each work out at our own pace but the company will be motivating.

Is there someone who can be a long-term eating-behavior partner? Yes. I have a friend with whom I've always been very open. She is not judgmental, and she has good insight into solving problems. I'm not embarrassed to tell her the things I eat or have problems with on a frequent basis. She also has a weight problem but does not get as obsessed with it as I do, but this may give me some balance in my approach.

How will I use that person to accomplish my long-term goals?
1. I'll tell her my weight on a weekly basis and make her promise that she won't let me stop doing this.
2. I'll call her when I feel like doing really compulsive eating or when I have been eating out of control for more than two days.
3. I'll let her advise me on what to do to get myself back on track, based on having already told her my goals.

29

You're Cured . . . Almost

*A*re you feeling good about your control? You should be, especially if you have worked on this for the past twenty-eight days. You can be proud of yourself if you feel in better control of your eating habits. It was hard work. You're probably even happier if you lost weight. That was hard work, too.

With hope, your good feeling will not turn into an invincible feeling. This chapter's title is designed to test you to see if you are feeling that control is yours for good. Even if you do not feel this way now, it is an important area to consider. If you continue to work hard on your eating habits, eventually there will be a period of time where it seems almost to come naturally. *Beware!* Do not get lulled into a false sense of security. It can be deadly to your good eating habits.

But don't let this discourage you. It is important that you feel that the control you have worked to build will continue to come more naturally without as much effort. And it will. But if you have struggled with your weight for any length of time, you must to some degree be aware of the failure rate of diets. And although this is not a diet, it is essential that you have ammunition to maintain your weight loss. Therefore, a first step is not getting too comfortable with your sense of control.

How do we get this idea that we are cured of our poor eating habits? Look back to another time when you were successful at losing weight. What happened to make you start to regain that weight? Following are some common pitfalls that you must now avoid in order to be successful permanently:

1. People tell you that you look wonderful. You probably don't see that as a negative. When people tell you how good you look, it certainly gives you a positive feeling. The problem is that frequently you get that feeling of invincibility that I mentioned previously. You may feel that if you look better, you must *be* better with your eating habits. The other thing this compliment does is to stop you short of your weight goal. Because you look so much better now and you receive all these compliments, you may ignore the fact that you have 15 more pounds to lose. Stopping short of your goal weight is a common cause of weight regain.

2. Not building a foundation. You must have a base upon which to build your eating habits. You must have a strong commitment to daily activities that will reinforce the positive changes you have made.

3. Getting away with things. There is frequently a period that follows controlled eating which we will call "test eating." This is a conscious or unconscious attempt to see how much you can get away with and still maintain your weight loss. The individual eats more then he is accustomed to and then weighs himself. "Good," he thinks, "I haven't gained any weight." Then he eats a little more, and if he gets by without the scale going up, he eats even more. This is a *big mistake*! There is often a lapse between food intake and weight gain. Sometimes this lapse is weeks long. During this time, you are returning to your old eating habits because you somehow think you can get away with it. Don't test your control. Stick with your new, good eating habits.

4. Going on a gimmick diet. I have written an entire book explaining why you should not diet at all but instead change your eating habits. Despite this fact, if you get into mild trouble in the future because those habits have waned a bit, don't give in to the temptation to try a gimmick diet. Doing so will not only result in a poor quality of weight loss, but you will likely regain it in a very short time.

You have now learned the basics to continue to lose weight if needed or to maintain that which you have already lost. Continuing to review these basics will help them to become almost second nature. Just remember that you must always be a bit more careful than other people with regard to your eating behavior.

Following are the nine most important points of this

book. They should already be ingrained in your mind, but if you've missed any of them, make a decision to learn them now and live by them. Try saying them aloud daily until they are a permanently a part of your mindset.

1. I will not think of my eating in black-and-white terms.
2. I will learn to do well 80 percent of the time, but I will take failure in stride when it happens.
3. I will limit my fat intake every way I can, also keeping calories in mind.
4. I will plan for snacks.
5. I will live by my "foundation."
6. I will eat 40 percent of my daily calories by 3:00 P.M.
7. I will exercise aerobically at least five days a week; three times will be between 4:00 and 6:00 P.M., before dinner.
8. I will engage in activities that make it more difficult to eat during the tough times.
9. I will continue to think of any plan that has even a remote chance of working to end snack attacks.

That's it. Those are the basics. Be careful, and don't get complacent. Also, don't get compulsively focused on control. Realize that 100 percent cured is not necessary; 80 percent will do.

Day 29 Assignment: You should be feeling good about your control over your eating habits by now. Take note of the nine most important points of this book, as listed above. Copy them in the space provided and read them aloud often.

WORKSHEET

Important points of this book

1. _____

2. _____

3. _____

4. _____

5. _____

6. _____

7. _____

8. _____

9. _____

30

A Form for
Forever Success

Day 30 Assignment: Well, this is it! Armed with good ammunition, you are on your own from here. Don't let down! Not even for a day. If necessary, reread this book every thirty days. The following will be the first of your monthly reviews to determine that your eating habits are on track. Talk to your partner today (if you have selected one) and make a plan of action for the next thirty days.

MONTHLY REVIEW FORM

Current weight_____ Goal weight_____
Weight at end of last month _____
Eating habits are _____ percent on track

SNACK ATTACK

Exercise habits are _____ percent on track

My foundation is:

1. _____

2. _____

3. _____

4. _____

5. _____

I am accomplishing these goals _____

percent of the time

I am doing well at _____

_____

My most difficult behavior currently is _____

_____

_____

To do better, I will _____

_____

_____

I will reward myself by _____

_____

A new improvement in my behavior by the end of next

month will be _____

_____